The L.O.V.E. Program: The Pathway to a Healthier You

THE DIET OF
L.O.V.E.

MORDECHAI S. NOSRATI, MD.

Associate Professor of Clinical Medicine
Keck USC School of Medicine

University of Southern California

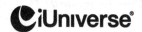

The Diet of L.O.V.E.
The L.O.V.E. Program: The Pathway to a Healthier You

iUniverse books may be ordered through booksellers or by contacting:

iUniverse
1663 Liberty Drive
Bloomington, IN 47403
www.iuniverse.com
1-800-Authors (1-800-288-4677)

ISBN: 978-1-4620-6042-9 (sc)
ISBN: 978-1-4620-6044-3 (hc)
ISBN: 978-1-4620-6043-6 (e)

Print information available on the last page.

iUniverse rev. date: 04/13/2016

Notice to the Reader

This book is intended as a reference volume only, not as a medical manual, guide, or replacement for a health-care provider.

The scientifically based information provided in this book is designed to help you make informed decisions about your health and nutrition. It is not intended as a replacement or substitute for any preventive measure or treatment that may have been prescribed by your physician or health-care provider. If you suspect that you have a medical condition or problem, I urge you to seek medical help immediately. In this comprehensive book, you will find many recommendations for supplements, minerals, vitamins, herbs, and other suggestions that will help you use these items safely and wisely. You should not start any exercise, physical fitness program, diet, or taking of dietary supplements without first consulting with a competent physician or health-care provider.

Internet addresses (URL) given in this book were accurate at the time it went to press.

This book is dedicated to my all-time teachers, my parents, to whom I owe all my yearnings and love for sciences and knowledge; to my wife, who has been always an inspiration to me; and last but not least, to all my teachers and professors throughout my education.

Contents

Physician's Daily Prayer

The almighty God of the universe, The Most High God, before I begin my holy duty, healing Your creation, I lay my supplication before You, that You will grant me the spirit, the strength and the enormous energy to do my work with faith, and that the desire to accumulate wealth would not blind my eyes from seeing one who is suffering, one who comes for my advice, as a human being, rich or poor, friend or foe, the good or the evil person, in his sorrowful moment reveal to me only the human being in him. My love for the learning of medicine should only strengthen my spirit; only the truth shall be the light before my feet, for any weakness in my work might bring about death and illness to your creation. I plead to you, please, merciful, compassionate, and gracious God, strengthen my body, my mind, and my soul and plant within me a spirit that is whole and holy. (Amen)

Maimonides, 1135–1204 CE

Preface

As a practicing physician, I have seen thousands of patients for more than two decades grapple with weight problems and their ensuing illnesses. Using a holistic approach to health, I have been successful in teaching my patients to change their lifestyle and behavior. After observing the effects of fad diets on different organs, and on the body systems as a whole, I decided to write this book to empower other individuals to change their eating habits. As a physician subspecializing in nephrology (study of the diseases of the kidneys) and internal medicine, I have dealt with the nutritional needs of critically ill and dialysis patients for many years. I have had the opportunity to interact with patients and with nutritionists. In addition, as an academician, teaching at Keck–USC School of Medicine, University of Southern California and its residence training program, I have taught interns, residents, and fellows for many years and have stressed the importance of nutrition in treating disease and promoting health.

One of the things I emphasize in discussing holistic health is that it is impossible to have a healthy body if what you eat is not healthy and balanced. "You are what you eat" is such a profound statement. Furthermore, nutrition is fuel for your body. I don't believe you would put low-grade or diesel fuel in your high-performance car engine. So, why would you poison yourself with poor and unbalanced nutrition?

A central component of practicing medicine, especially nephrology, is advocating proper nutrition. Nutrition is of paramount importance when taking care of severely ill patients. As a nephrologist and internist, I have been an adviser to nutrition departments and have helped formulate nutritional programs for a variety of patients, from the critically ill to the healthy ones who need to maintain their health status. In addition, because I am heavily involved in nutritional issues, my friends, relatives, and patients are constantly bombarding me with questions concerning popular fad diets and various diet programs. Through these close personal interactions, I have come to realize that people from all walks of life, including those one would consider well informed and educated, have difficulty not only choosing the right diet but following it as well. They are doing fanatical and extreme things to lose weight, thus putting themselves in great harm physiologically and psychologically.

Another major motivation for writing this book is that as a nephrologist, I can bear witness to the devastating effects of kidney disease, heart disease, and diabetes mellitus. Every day I see patients on dialysis and observe the overall suffering it causes. Currently, more than three hundred fifty thousand people are on dialysis. It is estimated that by 2010, there will be six hundred thousand people on some form of dialysis (see note 1). We all know the economic burden that kidney disease and dialysis care has placed on society but that topic is outside the scope of this book.

I wrote this book to encourage and assist people who blindly follow these dangerous and unhealthy fad diets. These fad diets (e.g., Atkins diet, Protein Power, the Zone, South Beach, and Sugar Busters) can put an enormous stress on the kidneys and the body as a whole (see notes 2–11). I am hopeful that with publication of this book, which is full of simple ideas for weight loss, I will be able to help many people achieve their ultimate goal of weight loss without jeopardizing their health. Via this program, I educate people about a more holistic approach to health and well-being, emphasizing good nutrition, a healthy mind, and spiritual enrichment.

It is my contention that a healthy eating guide must be based on the latest and most sound scientific evidence. I strove to do so without making this book too complicated for easy reading. I will give you the latest information on new discoveries that should have profound effects on our eating patterns. This diet does not restrict a lot of food categories and does not believe in starvation. Hopefully, it will be a successful plan that you will adhere to for years.

I seek to make good nutrition a simple thing and a fun thing for everyone, so it becomes a part of your daily life and routine. In a fast-paced society such as ours, it is very difficult and time consuming to go to the gym every day. If you are able to do that, I tip my hat to you, and I hope you continue. Since you are, ultimately, what you eat, I emphasize good nutrition and by this, teach you to make better choices about what you eat. I present a whole new approach to a healthier you. The approach is holistic, incorporating a mind-body-spirit experience. Diet, physical activity, relaxation and stress-reduction techniques, and spirituality are encouraged, and we will see the interconnectedness of these components toward maintaining sound health. Also, I emphasize that fact that you are a composition of a physical body, a powerful mind, and a beautiful soul. After all, we human beings are complex. I believe it is a great injustice to be dealt with as just a number, a name, and a simple physical being. I always approach my patients, whether in the intensive care unit or in the office, as a combination of mind, body, and soul. I can prescribe the most potent medications to treat physical ailments, but if the patient is suffering from emotional or psychological issues, medications alone are not the answer.

We are great spirits in a material world full of emotions. We live in such a quick-fix society that many of us are brainwashed into the "crash diet approach" to weight loss. We live in such a materialistic world that we have lost contact with our inner self and, as such, are constantly striving to find happiness based on material wealth. It is never too late to get in touch with your inner self. Develop the spiritual enrichment that lies within you. Let's start now!

Mordechai S. Nosrati MD Feb 18, 2016

Disclaimer

This book provides scientific information on health aspects of micronutrients and phytochemicals for the general public. The information is made available with the understanding that the author is not providing medical, psychological, or nutritional counseling services in this book and on its sites. The information should not be used in place of a consultation with a competent health-care or nutrition professional.

The information contained in this book and its website does not cover all possible uses, actions, precautions, side effects, and interactions. It is not intended as medical advice for individual problems. Liability for individual actions or omissions based on the contents of this site is expressly disclaimed.

Introduction

L.O.V.E. Diet Program

My L.O.V.E. diet is a program with a unique, wholesome approach to the big epidemic that plagues our society—obesity. In this work, I bring together the mind-body-soul experience with the scientifically proven aspects of the DASH diet, with an emphasis on a healthier Mediterranean diet. A healthier and wholesome combination of fruits and vegetables, with animal protein in moderation was taught centuries ago by the prominent Jewish scholar, philosopher, and physician Maimonides. *The Diet of L.O.V.E.* also encompasses several other well-balanced diets. However, as society became more industrialized and the need for processing and preservation of food became necessary to feed many people away from home, healthier diets were replaced by unhealthy processed foods.

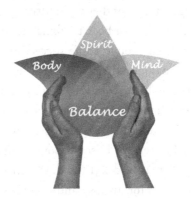

A Mind-Body-Spirit Experience

It is critical, and logical, that you approach any goal that you set for yourself in life as a mind-body-spirit experience. After all, you are a combination of these three interconnected, interdependent, and inseparable components. It is impossible to concentrate on one component and let go of the others.

You cannot just take care of the physical body without giving attention to your mind and your soul. If these components are disconnected, you as an individual are not at peace and in balance. Imagine that you are stressed about an interview or an exam. You can feel the effect of this emotional stress as indigestion, irritable bowels, or other symptoms—a mind-over-body effect. Hence, it is absolutely impossible to disconnect these components, and attempts to do so will fail. It is a significant point that needs to be addressed, learned, and understood by every person who wishes to improve his or her life, including diet.

You should always regard your body as a sacred temple, and as such, your body is the temple of God and should be looked after. Within this temple rests your inner soul, the divine extension of the infinite God. Doesn't that beautiful inner soul desire a well-nourished and healthy place to rest in order to manifest its full potentials and hidden powers?

Fad Diets: Think Before You Dive In!

The number of people on a diet has increased dramatically in the last few years. A new national survey indicates that one-third of adult Americans, or seventy-one million, are currently on a diet—an increase of 35 percent since 2000 (see note 12). This is the highest level of dieting in fifteen years, according to the Calorie Control Council, which has been tracking dieting and weight control habits since 1984 (13). Even though some succeed in losing the weight, a greater percentage fail to maintain their weight loss and regain the weight lost and even more. Obesity and being overweight in the United States has been on the rise and has become a major public-health problem. By some estimates, more than 40 percent of Americans are considered overweight. Overweight has been defined by the Centers for Disease Control and Prevention (CDC) as people who have a body mass index (BMI) between 25 and 29.9 (14). This has led our society to search for an easy and effortless way to lose weight, kind of a "magic bullet" to help us lose weight quickly and effortlessly. But almost all these fad diets are full of empty promises and are usually not free from health dangers, not to mention the emotional impacts that these fad diets and failure to achieve the desired weight have on your self-esteem and confidence! In addition, your emotional state of mind also becomes tremendously altered, often causing you to become depressed at times.

Fad diets are temporary and short-lived approaches to weight loss; they don't work over the long haul. These diets promise results they can't deliver. Food choices are often not balanced, and the caloric intakes are very restricted. These diets are like time bombs that can jeopardize your health at any time.

The most popular diets are those that promote low carbohydrate and high protein intake and promise significant weight loss. These diets are typical low-calorie diets in disguise, but with some potentially serious consequences.

Atkins Diet and Its Health Concerns

The health concerns of Atkins and other high-protein fad diets include increased rate of colon cancer, increased risk of cardiovascular disease, decreased kidney function, increased formation of kidney stones, and osteoporosis.

These fad diets and programs, especially Atkins diet, emphasize an intake of large amounts of meat, fats, and dairy products that are loaded with cholesterol, saturated fat, and animal protein.

The American Heart Association, American Dietetic Association, and the American Kidney Fund have all published position papers warning people of the health hazards and various dangers associated with low-carbohydrate, high-protein diets (2, 3, 13). The health dangers of the Atkins diet are numerous. People who pursue these crazed and unbalanced diets are consequently at risk for deficiencies in vitamin and mineral intake, as well as potential cardiac, renal, bone, and liver abnormalities.

A clinical study showed that high-protein diets may cause permanent loss of kidney function in anyone with already reduced kidney function (15). In addition, other studies have shown a strong association between diets with a heavy intake of meat and a significant increase in the risk for colon cancer and osteoporosis (16). As for the calcium losses on high-protein diets (i.e., Atkins diet), it can reach, on average, 50 to 60 percent above normal (17). These heavy losses of calcium can severely affect population at risk for osteoporosis and ultimately increase the rate of bone and hip fractures.

It is now evident from some studies that in the short term, you can lose weight on the Atkins diet. In reality, any diet can make you lose some weight in the beginning. But what the Atkins diet proposes is the worst and most dangerous diet for the long term. Dieters following this fad will pay for this skewed and irresponsible diet with their health. In my opinion, the Atkins diet is the most unbalanced and unhealthy diet plan out there. This diet can wreak havoc on your cardiovascular and skeletal system, not to mention increase risk of certain cancers (18–22).

Proponents and promoters of the Atkins diet falsely claim that diets low in carbohydrates force the body to turn to other fuels for energy and that cutting out carbohydrate-containing foods will lead to weight loss. Therefore, they claim that due to the lack of carbohydrates, the body attempts to get energy from fats and proteins in the diet or from body fat itself.

It is a misconception that only carbohydrate-rich foods are the cause of obesity. Several clinical trials and large epidemiological studies on Asian and Mediterranean people have shown that people who consume a large amount of carbohydrates in the form of rice, noodles, and vegetables in general have lower body weights compared to Americans (23, 24). This fact even holds true after they have immigrated to the United States. For example, Asian Americans who eat large amounts of meat, dairy products, and carbohydrates are generally still not as heavy as Americans (24).

Low-carbohydrate diets characteristically include cholesterol, fat, saturated fat, and protein that exceed the recommended daily allowances and current dietary guidelines. They are certainly very low in fiber and other important dietary ingredients. Therefore, it is a fact that high-protein diets restrict healthful foods that provide essential nutrients for a healthy body and adequate nutrition. Similarly, vegetarians, who generally follow diets rich in carbohydrates foods, typically have significantly lower body weights than omnivores. These vegetarians who have a lower body weight likely consume more complex carbohydrates than simple carbohydrates, which are the culprits in many diets.

As stated previously, high-protein diets cause deterioration of kidney functioning (15, 16). It is important to point out that the kidney-damaging effects were seen only with animal proteins, and no harmful effects were seen with plant proteins. It is estimated that as many as 20 to 25 percent of adults in the United States may suffer from reduced kidney functioning without even being aware of it. The percentage is drastically higher for people over forty, diabetics, or hypertensive individuals. For example, mild to moderate kidney disease is found in 40 percent of diabetics! In fact, it is estimated that kidney disease and requirements for dialysis will be the next epidemic in the United States (25, 26). The fact that people who have kidney problems are unaware of them complicates this epidemic. With the introduction of high-protein diets, these people in particular will be at greater risk for further worsening of kidney functioning.

People who have followed the high-protein diets have reported other side effects, such as constipation (more than 65 percent), headache (about 60 percent), halitosis or bad breath (about 35 percent), and general weakness (25 percent) (27). These and other dangers have been reported and discussed about other fad diets that are promoted on the radio, TV, and billboards, and in magazines, diet books, and other media outlets. These dangers are more pronounced, since the media pressure to diet has significantly increased over the past thirty years, bombarding us like never before.

Last but Not Least: Liposuction's Risks and Dangers

Liposuction is a surgical procedure, and it is not risk free. The risks and complications of liposuction range from mild to potentially life threatening. The risks increase with the number of areas to be treated, the amount of fat removed, and the length of the surgery.

The risks involved with liposuction procedures include contour irregularities, scars, numbness and tingling, organ failure, shock and death from fat and blood embolization (formation and passage of blood clots to the lungs), and infections. It may be necessary to remove excess skin after a liposuction, putting the individual at risk for more surgical complications.

It is also important to remember that patients who are immunocompromised or suffer from diabetes, poor blood circulation, or heart or lung disease should not undergo liposuction without a careful evaluation and supervision of medical specialists due to unacceptable higher risk of developing life-threatening infections and non-healing wounds.

Major Risks Associated with Liposuction

| Infection |
| Prolonged healing time |
| Reaction to anesthesia |
| Embolization to the lungs |
| Shock |
| Damage to the skin or nerves |
| Organ failure |
| Death |

Now before starting the discussion and teachings of the Diet of L.O.V.E, you need to be introduced to the very important requirements and components of this "way of L.O.V.E." What I am referring to are the "Ten Commandments" of L.O.V.E. which are essential for achieving the important and healthy goals intended by this multifaceted "scientific" and "holistic" approach to a whole new way of achieving the optimal health and weight management.

Chapter One

My L.O.V.E. Diet Program and Its Commandments

The Ten Commandments of L.O.V.E.

I. Thou shalt love yourself.
II. Thou shalt love others.
III. Thou shalt nourish your soul.
IV. Thou shalt nourish your body.
V. Thou shalt nourish your mind.
VI. Thou shalt forgive others.
VII. Thou shalt set reasonable goals.
VIII. Thou shalt have a positive outlook.
IX. Thou shalt reduce stress.
X. Thou shalt increase your physical activity.

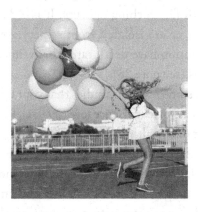

I. Thou Shalt Love Yourself

The Holy Bible teaches a very profound commandment, "Love your neighbor as yourself." This is not a selfless love. In reality, this commandment attempts to emphasize that loving yourself is a good thing and that this love should be extended to others. If you do not love yourself, how will you possibly love your neighbor?

If you see yourself as an inadequate, ugly, or inept person, others will see you that way too. If you put yourself down, how can you expect others to respect you? If you fail to truly love yourself, how can you ever learn to love anyone else?

That is why learning to love yourself is the greatest love of all. How do we learn to love ourselves? You have to truly believe in the concept of being created in the image of God. You have a purpose and destiny in this life.

The real reason to learn to love yourself is to reach beyond yourself, to use your love of self to then love others, even strangers, and, ultimately, all of humanity.

Loving Yourself and Your Health

An integral part of any successful diet is that you should truly love yourself. As soon as you reach this essential stage, the effort that is required to take care of your body and diet needs will no longer be an uphill struggle but a natural desire to take good care of yourself.

Love and health are very closely related. The commandment of "Love thy neighbor" is not just an ethical command but also a physical and physiological one with far-reaching benefits. It is a documented fact that people who live alone or are isolated from society are more predisposed to illness—not to mention have death rates three times higher than more socially active persons (see note 28).

It is evident from some research studies that your body, brain, and mind respond positively when you experience love (29–31). Love appears to be the important ingredient of a healthy body and mind.

Close personal relationships have the ability to reduce stress. When you are in a close relationship, you feel less threatened, more confident, supported, and ultimately, more in control. It is evident that when you feel supported, you have feelings of security, optimism, and hope. This is a great stress reducer, so love yourself and love others. It is good for you!

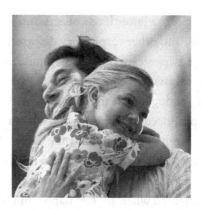

II. Thou Shalt Love Others

When you feel love and compassion, it boosts your immune system. Many research studies demonstrate that love does indeed improve our health (32–38). These studies look at love, loving, and being in love. Feeling loved seems to benefit our cardiovascular health and its disease outcome. Giving love seems to do the same thing for the aging process; it slows the physiology of aging and illness. Studies on aging have shown that the effects of aging were influenced more by what people contribute to society than what they received from it. Simply, the more love and support you give, the more you experience the anti-aging effects of love.

Social ties at every level—from close family to coworkers and community—that involve love and intimacy of any type may also boost your immune system and, thereby, protect you against infectious diseases. When you feel loved, cared for, supported, or intimate, you are most likely to be happier and healthier. You will have a better immune system, with a much lower risk of getting sick. Furthermore, if you do get seriously ill, you will have a much greater chance of surviving. Researchers have discovered that when you feel love or, in fact, experience any positive emotion, such as compassion, caring, or gratitude, the heart sends messages to the brain and hormones are released that positively affect your health (35–38).

It has been shown that when you feel and remain angry for short periods of time, as short as five minutes, your cortisol level in your blood increases (39). Cortisol, a stress hormone, suppresses the immune system. Studies have shown that this rise in cortisol level after feeling angry suppresses the formation of certain antibodies (IgA, immunoglobulin A) for five to six hours (39). These antibodies are your body's first line of defense against infection and disease. So, the lower levels of IgA antibodies leave you more vulnerable to colds, flu, and other respiratory diseases. On the other hand, when you feel loved and appreciated for five minutes, your IgA antibodies rise significantly, which lasts for many hours.

Endorphins are endogenous materials that have morphine-like properties. They are produced in major organs of your body, including the brain, genitalia, gut, immune system, and the heart. Some studies have shown that endorphins, which are associated with the feeling of ecstasy, help you bond and form loving relationships with other people. Simply put, endorphins are released when we feel happy and loved. They can also stimulate natural killer cells, the special immune system cells that fight precancer cells, cancerous cells and tumors, and virus-infected cells in addition to orchestrating innate immunity of the organism.

It is interesting to note that to reap the benefits of love, you need not have a lover or spouse. The love you feel can be for anyone: a parent, a child, a sibling, or even a coworker. In fact, this love can even be toward a pet or even plants. A large body of evidence supports the fact that you will have a better outcome in a major illness or surgery if you own a pet. This fact is more evident and marked in elderly patients (40, 41). One can speculate that because elderly so often have lost many of their friends and family members, they would benefit from the close companionship of animals.

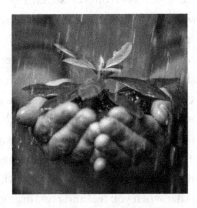

III. Thou Shalt Nourish Your Soul

You are not just your physical body but also your mind and your soul. So, get in touch with that inner soul and nourish it. Reach for that inner spirit that lies within you and cherish it. Remember, you are divine.

You are divine and can reach many goals in your life with the help of this divine source within you. We are not just a mere collection of trillions of cells. The spirit and the breath of God—the infinite—lie within you. You can achieve wonders, since you are a part of the infinite. So, nourish your soul as you nourish your physical body. Live the mind-body-spirit experience.

Spirituality and Health

In ancient times, mind, body, and soul were seen as interconnected and inseparable from physical health. Spirituality and health were seen as inseparable, closely attached, and interwoven entities. Simply put, if one element in this whole were to be disturbed, all other parts would be affected.

How spirituality influences health was not known until recent discoveries and research. However, it appeared to our ancestors that the body, mind, and soul (spirit) are somehow connected and interact. The health status of each of these elements appears to affect the others as if they are inseparable.

Research has discovered that the bond, comfort, support, and strength achieved from religion, meditation, and prayer can influence the healing and health of the individual (42–45). Spirituality can, by no means, cure an illness (at least no one has proven it), but it can help you adapt and deal with the illness and its ramifications.

Spirituality means different things to different people. Spirituality can be defined as the way you find and bring meaning, hope, support, comfort, and inner peace into your life. You may find tranquility, which some people equate with spirituality, through religion, philosophy, art, music, or being in harmony with nature. Almost all religions of the world emphasize the concept of spirituality.

Spiritual people may live longer and healthier lives than others, according to research studies (42–45). People who describe themselves as moderately spiritual are, in general, healthier than those who report low levels of spirituality. It is evident that any level of spirituality provides an edge to those who practice it through the health benefits of reduced stress and healthier lifestyles—all of which are known factors in lowering mortality.

To have a healthy body, you must have a healthy mind and a spirited soul that can influence and support each other in times of trouble. In our demanding and fast-paced society, where everything has turned to numbers and images without any spiritual significance, it is imperative to bring in each of these three elements—body, mind, and soul—to work in concert to assist you in achieving in your work and goals. One excellent way to nourish the mind and to become more aware of the links between mind, body, and soul is to practice meditation.

Meditation

Many ancient religious sects have incorporated the practice of meditation (in one form or another) into their services to bring a harmony between mind and body, and ultimately, soul and body. After all, several major religions hold the premise that we are born in the image of God, and a sparkle of God resides deep inside each one of us. We are more than just a mere physical body.

The use of meditation for healing and improving physical and mental health is nothing new. Meditative techniques are diverse, because of the influences of varied cultures and religious groups around the globe.

More physicians and health-care providers prescribe meditation as a way to lessen anxiety and depression, lower blood pressure, improve breathing and sense of well-being, relieve insomnia, and as an overall means to combat the everyday stresses of life. In fact, the importance of meditation to lessen suffering and promote healing was understood and practiced for centuries in advanced ancient cultures, such as Jews (kabbalists), Chinese, Hindus, and Indians (46–49).

Meditation is extremely safe and doesn't require much technique or equipment. It can be performed almost anywhere. All you need to meditate is to close your eyes and "mindscape" to everything around you. Then, concentrate on the inner part of you, and look for and get in touch with that inner self that exists apart from one's reactions to daily life. This can be done for as little as a minute up to hours. Remember, it is very simple and can benefit anybody.

Research studies have shown that meditation can produce a state of deep relaxation (50–52). This deep relaxation is evidenced by multiple physiological markers, such as decreased heart rate, decreased respiratory rate, and decreased blood cortisol level. The effect of meditation is so strong that it can affect the brain activity as documented by alpha waves seen on an EEG—a brain wave that is present in the deep state of relaxation.

Research has also discovered that with meditation, your brain becomes more alert, and your mind can react much faster and with greater creativity and comprehension. On the other hand, the body feels rested as a result of meditation. Meditation also has other effects on the activities of the nervous system. In fact, the parasympathetic nervous system—which makes a person feel calm—dominates.

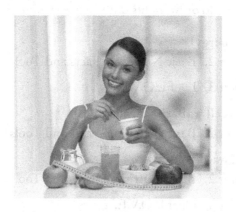

IV. Thou Shalt Nourish Your Body

Body Nourishment

A well-nourished body helps you achieve and maintain a healthy weight and have enough energy and vitality for daily physical activities. Good nutrition is directly related to health and the prevention of many diseases, as well as a key factor in well-being. Food, water, and sleep are all critical parts of nourishing the body. Nourishment of your physical body is accomplished through a well-balanced and healthy diet. The basic principles of healthy nutrition are a balanced meal and eating in moderation. Simply put, you are what you eat. A healthy and well-balanced meal calls for a wide variety of nutrients, minerals, and vitamins. So, nourish your body!

Major Nutrients Your Body Needs

+ Carbohydrates
+ Proteins

- Fats
- Fiber
- Vitamins and minerals
- Water

Major Nutrients and Their Function

Carbohydrates (energy)
- See chapter 2, "Basic Nutrition: Facts and Tools"
- See chapter 3, "L. of L.O.V.E."

Proteins (energy, cell wall, tissue, enzymes)
- See chapter 2, "Basic Nutrition: Facts and Tools"

Fats (energy, cell wall)
- See chapter 2, "Basic Nutrition: Facts and Tools"
- See chapter 4, "O. of L.O.V.E."

Fiber (function of gut)
- See chapter 2, "Basic Nutrition: Facts and Tools"
- See chapter 3, "L. of L.O.V.E."

Vitamins and minerals (metabolism, cell functions)
- See chapter 2, "Basic Nutrition: Facts and Tools"

Water (metabolism, waste, cell functions)
- See chapter 2, "Basic Nutrition: Facts and Tools"
- See chapter 9, "Detoxification: A Simple Preparation for a Healthy Body"

Pure and Refreshing Water

Water makes up 50 to 60 percent of the human body. It is extremely important to drink an adequate amount of water as part of a healthy diet. Water nourishes the body, and proper hydration helps each cell to function properly. Drinking adequate amounts of water facilitates blood circulation to the major organs, thereby helping them function properly. It is vital to your survival. There's no substitute for water!

Water regulates body temperature and blood circulation, cushions joints, and protects tissues and organs—including the spinal cord—from shock and damage. In addition to carrying nutrients and oxygen to cells, water removes toxins and other waste products. Lack of water, dehydration, can cause many ailments, including hypertension, asthma, allergies, and migraine headaches.

You should drink at least eight to ten eight-ounce glasses of water each day as part of a healthy diet. Drink water throughout the day rather than only when thirsty. Of course, if your physician places you on a special water restriction, you should follow it strictly.

Water and Weight Loss

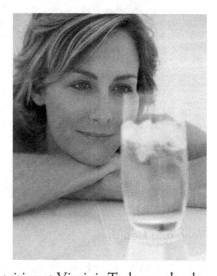

Drinking water may be the most important piece of the weight-loss puzzle. Water contains no calories, fat, or cholesterol and is low in sodium. It is nature's appetite suppressant and helps the body to metabolize fat. It is believed low water intake yields an increase in fat deposits (468, 469). Conversely, high water intake reduces the amount fat deposits. Research suggests that drinking plenty of water may help you lose weight. In a study by Dr. Brenda Davy, associate professor of human nutrition at Virginia Tech, people who drank two glasses of water approximately thirty minutes before every meal lost weight more quickly initially and lost significantly more weight than those who didn't. In another study by the same group of researchers, Dr. Davy found that people who drank water before meals consumed an average of seventy-five fewer calories at that meal! To a layperson, this may not seem like much, however, if you eat seventy-five fewer calories during each meal (breakfast, lunch, and dinner) for the whole year, you can lose about twenty-one pounds! In addition, being even 1 percent dehydrated can cause a significant drop in metabolism, which can also interfere with weight loss (471–480). Without enough water, the kidneys cannot function properly.

As a result, some of their workload is pushed off onto the liver, preventing it from operating at peak levels (53).

How does all this tie into weight loss? Because metabolizing fat is a primary function of the liver, and because the liver can't function at peak levels when taking on added workload from the kidneys, less body fat is metabolized and more is stored. This leads to either weight gain or reaching a plateau of weight loss. When dieting, we restrict the calories we take in, to some degree. By doing so, we lessen the total amount of water available to our bodies, since about 30 percent of the average person's water intake comes from the food they eat. This gives us even more reason to raise our water intake.

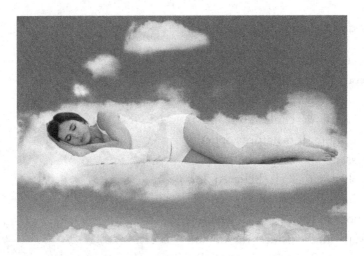

Sleep and Health

To stay healthy, your body requires "down time" to not rest and repair itself. The best way to accomplish this is to ensure enough sleep hours daily.

Sleep is a major and unavoidable component of basic human physiology. It is extremely essential for a healthier and higher quality of life. You sleep almost a third of your life. On average, most people need approximately eight hours of sleep a night. However, this can vary greatly between four hours and ten hours for different people. It is evident that good quality sleep is essential for your well-being and health.

Sleep, and lack of it, can affect your performance during the day. You most likely have experienced the fact that when you don't get enough sleep, your concentration, effectiveness, and energy level decline the next day.

Cortisol dictates when your body should be active and when it should rest. Cortisol levels in your blood follow the circadian rhythm (a twenty-four-hour cycle). It peaks as the sun rises and dips as the sun sets. When the cortisol levels rise, you feel more energetic to start your day. Three to four hours after dark, your cortisol levels dip low and reach their nadir; your body enters into a period of rest, recuperation, and recovery. However, many lifestyle and environmental factors can cause difficulties in sleeping.

According to some researchers, sleep serves many purposes in both humans and animals. Apparently, animals sleep to regulate body temperature, organize memories, and replenish the immune system. The cells, organs, hormones, and immune factors in the body, like the brain, may contain molecular clocks that help drive daily sleep and wake cycles (54).

Inadequate rest impairs the ability to think, handle stress, and maintain a healthy immune system. In animal studies, total sleep deprivation is fatal in some species (55). It has long been known that total sleep deprivation is 100 percent lethal to rats; however, on autopsy, the animals look completely normal. It is evident that the rats develop bacterial infections of the blood, as if their immune systems had crashed. In another study, healthy men and women were deprived of sleep for three days while their blood was monitored for immune system factors. Researchers expected to see a decline in immune function, yet the opposite happened: the subjects' immune systems were overactive (56)! The main effects of sleep deprivation include sleepiness, fatigue, stress, and deterioration of performance, attention, and motivation (56).

A German study lends strong support to the notion that creativity and problem solving appear to be directly linked to adequate sleep (57). Additionally, they have demonstrated that your sleeping brain continues working on problems that confound you during the day, and the right answer may come more easily after eight hours of rest. These findings provide a valuable reminder to people who are overtired and to overburdened students that sleep is often the best medicine.

Make sure that you get enough sleep every day. If you are chronically tired, fatigued, and mentally slow all the time, you will be surprised at how much more energetic and sharp you will feel once you start sleeping normally. Getting a good night's sleep is critical to your health and well-being.

Lack of Sleep and Weight Gain

A mounting body of research connects inadequate sleep and the increased risk of a number of health conditions, such as type II diabetes, hypertension, and obesity (58). Onaverage, Americans today are getting less sleep than they did a century ago. Interestingly, with declining sleep time, there has also been an increase in obesity in the United States.

Researchers have found that there is an inverse relationship between total sleep time and index of obesity (59). As the total sleep time decreased, their patients' body mass index (BMI) increased, except in the severely obese subjects. In other words, obese and overweight patients sleep less than people with medically defined normal body weight (normal BMI).

A strong association has been shown scientifically, through epidemiology, between the amount of sleep you get and the risk of gaining weight and becoming obese (58). People who get fewer than four hours of sleep a night are more likely to be obese than those who get seven to nine hours of rest. The risk of obesity decreases by 20 percent for each hour of extra sleep.

Given the fact that you burn fewer calories when you are resting, it may seem counterintuitive and absurd that sleeping more would prevent obesity, though it's true you don't eat while asleep. There is scientific evidence that demonstrates a link between sleep and the various central nervous system pathways that regulate food intake (59). Also, chronic sleep deprivation may have some effect on your brain's food-seeking behavior, possibly in an attempt to gain energy.

Clearly, sleep deprivation lowers leptin, a protein that suppresses appetite. Leptin affects how your brain senses whether you have had enough food. Sleep deprivation also raises levels of a substance that makes you want to eat more. This substance is called grehlin.

Another pivotal study has shown that even in otherwise healthy young people, a sleep debt of three or four hours a night over the course of a week can affect the body's ability to process carbohydrates. Another major study found that lack of sleep at a younger age in men could suppress the production of growth hormones later in life. Growth hormones play an essential role during adulthood in controlling the body's proportions of fat and muscle. Therefore, lower growth hormone levels in younger years increase the tendency to become overweight later in life (60–64).

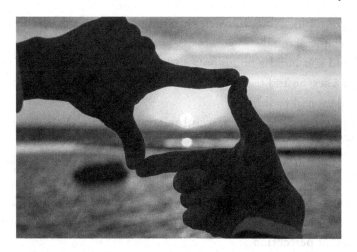

V. Thou Shalt Have a Positive Attitude

"You are your thoughts; the rest of you are bones and fiber. If you think of roses, you are a rose garden; if you think of thorns, you are fuel for the furnace" (Jalaludin Rumi).

Positive thinking and a positive attitude are pivotal to achieving any goal in life— whether big or small. Never underestimate the power of your mind in any aspect of your life, from your career to your relationships and your health, to how you perceive and view situations in life and the world in general. Whether you are optimistic or pessimistic will determine and influence the outcome. If you approach life with a positive attitude and perspective, it will influence the outcome. Your attitude will influence what direction your life will take.

Two patients with the same illness who receive the same treatment may not fare the same. The one who is optimistic and positive will fare better than the one who is pessimistic and negative. The optimistic patient is in a better state of mind and is more likely to follow the doctor's orders. In addition, positive feelings can affect the immune system. Our words, our thoughts, and our attitudes create and form our reality. A positive attitude, combined with optimistic words and thoughts, creates a positive world for us to live in. Positive attitude and thinking can influence the outcome of your endeavors. So, live in a prosperous and tranquil state—beautiful mindscape. A mindscape is what you create for yourself, your own world. In your mind, you can reach beyond the stars and go to the depth of the seas. In your mind, you can reach anyone and go anywhere you desire. So, set your frame of mind.

Would you build a house on a garbage dump? Or would you build a house in a serene and tranquil atmosphere? Your soul and your mind are the foundation of your life.

Set your mindscape in a peaceful and tranquil state! Be at peace within yourself.

In a tranquil mind, your pains are not as noxious, and your joys are more pronounced. Imagine you won one million dollars ten minutes ago. Would you perceive a toothache the same? Or can a headache feel like it can be dealt with much easier? However you perceive a situation, the situation becomes that perception.

Be grateful, and attract good vibes into your life. Know that you are blessed, and see the abundance of it all around you. Be filled with happiness, and be thankful for what you have. Spend ten minutes a day in meditation.

"The secret of achievement is to hold a picture of a successful outcome in mind" (Henry David Thoreau, Poet and Philosopher).

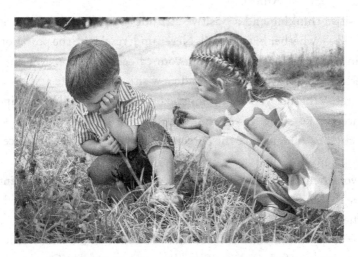

VI. Thou Shalt Forgive Others

We all carry baggage from our past, and this baggage gets heavier and heavier as we travel down the road of life. Our subconscious is bombarded by unpleasant and unresolved life experiences. These experiences can haunt us for the rest of our lives, unless we deal with them. The best and easiest way to do so is probably to forgive those who have hurt us. It is very important to note that we can be hurt by almost anyone, even the ones who truly love us. And if you think we can avoid being hurt, you must live in seclusion.

Forgiving is not an easy feat. In fact, it can be extremely difficult for some of us. It is obvious that the harder it is for you to forgive, the more chronic medical problems—such as high blood pressure, heart problems, stress, depression, and other mental conditions—you may experience (65).

So, drop the baggage and open it up. Resolve and discard the dirty laundry. Keep the weight of your baggage to a minimum; it will hold you back in life and stop you from doing the things you enjoy. Try hard to forgive others as well as yourself. Remember the concept of loving yourself. Forgiveness can be a powerful way to resolve this. It may take you a while to let go of things, but start now. Forgiveness is divine, and we, in striving to reach spirituality, have to emulate our creator. So, forgive and start living. A major component of forgiving is to show your compassion, so let your compassion shine through.

You may ask what forgiveness can accomplish. The act of forgiveness is divine, but it has an important connection to our physical well-being. Forgiveness is typically defined as the process of concluding resentment, indignation, or anger as a result of a perceived offense, difference, or mistake, and/or ceasing to demand punishment or restitution (66).

In the past few decades, the concept of forgiveness, which had been a practice of faith and religion, has been dealt with in the field of psychology. However, even though there is no current consensus on the psychological definition of "forgiveness" in the medical literature, some agreement has emerged via a number of published models describing the process of forgiveness (67).

There is a general path people follow when they forgive someone who has unjustly injured them. This process is not a rigid sequence, and individuals may experience all or only some of the steps. The process of forgiveness is mainly divided in four phases. Phase 1 is the uncovering phase, during which the individual becomes aware of the emotional pain that has resulted from a deep, unjust injury. Phase 2 is the decision phase, in which the individual realizes that to continue to focus on the injury and the injurer may cause more unnecessary suffering. Phase 3 is the work phase, when the individual begins the active work of forgiving the injurer. This phase may include new ways of thinking about the injurer. During the fourth phase, the outcome/deepening phase, the forgiving individual begins to realize that she or he is gaining emotional relief from the process of forgiving the injurer.

One of the more detailed studies on the effects of forgiveness was performed by Professor Robert Enright, founder of the International Forgiveness Institute. He has developed the 20-Step Process Model of Forgiveness (68). Some of his work has focused on what kind of person is more likely to be forgiving. A longitudinal study showed that people who were generally more neurotic, angry, and hostile were less likely to forgive another person even after a long time had passed. Particularly, these people were more likely to avoid the people who had hurt them and want to act out "payback" or retribution on them even four and a half years after the wrongdoing (69).

Some studies show that people who forgive are not only happier but also healthier than those who hold resentment and bitterness (65). For example, one of the earliest studies that looked at the way the act of forgiveness improves physical health discovered that when people think about forgiving an offender, it leads to improved cardiovascular and nervous system functioning (70). Meanwhile, another study discovered that the more forgiving the individual, the less likely the person was to suffer from many illnesses. On the other hand, the less forgiving individuals reported a greater number of health problems (71).

It is interesting to note that according to some research studies, the act of forgiveness can be learned (72). For example, in three unrelated studies, it was shown that individuals who are taught how to forgive get less angry, feel less hurt, become more optimistic, are more likely to be more forgiving in a variety of circumstances, and grow to be more compassionate and self-confident (70–74). Other studies show a reduction in stress and its physical manifestations and an increase in vitality (73).

When you honestly forgive people who have done you wrong, you let go of the negative and stressful feelings associated with those unpleasant events. This will probably increase the chances of loving one another and perhaps strengthen your relationships. *Don't forget about self-forgiveness.* Let go of your guilty feelings, and don't let them drag you down. Recognize your mistakes, and learn from them.

Forgiveness and Health

Complementary to the above evidence, scientists have discovered that when you forgive easily, you benefit from a better physical and mental health in contrast to those who carry grudges. In addition, you will have a lower rate of anxiety and depression. So, let go of those bad feelings, it is good for you.

People who are unable to forgive have higher blood pressure rates, more tension, and an overall higher stress level—no matter how trivial or unpleasant the incident. There is plenty of evidence to show that emotionally significant experiences tend to be well remembered (74, 75). This fact is evident from our own personal experiences as well as from extensive research findings. Significant experiences such as birthdays, wedding or graduation ceremonies, or the loss of a loved one characteristically leave lasting and dramatic memories. The conclusions of some research studies indicate that individuals have excellent recollections of where they were and what they were doing when they experienced earthquakes (76) or witnessed accidents (77).

Likewise, in animal studies involving rats, the animal remembers the place in an apparatus where it received an electrical shock or the position of an escape platform in a container filled with water (78, 79). Interestingly, these memory enhancements are not limited to unpleasant or traumatic experiences; pleasurable events also tend to be well remembered.

Extensive evidence indicates that stress hormones (epinephrine, glucocorticoids) released from the adrenal glands are critically involved in memory consolidation of emotionally arousing experiences. These stress hormones administered after exposure to emotionally arousing experiences enhance the consolidation of long-term memories of these experiences (80–83).

Therefore, it is not surprising that even past unpleasant experiences are as harmful as new ones. People who hold on to bad experiences from the distant past experience these unpleasant physiological effects every time they remember them (84). In contrast, people who forgive have reduced blood pressure and fewer heart problems.

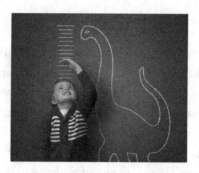

VII. Thou Shalt Set Reasonable Goals

You should not attempt to lose weight too rapidly. Set goals that are reachable, and when you reach the goals, set new ones. You should keep track of your pounds lost and reward yourself when you reach your goals. For example, keep track of the money that you would have spent on junk food, fast food, snacks, and high-calorie drinks, and reward yourself with perfume, cologne, clothing, or a spa treatment.

Set short- and long-term goals. Success will provide you with a sense of satisfaction. Try to incorporate those goals into your daily routine. When setbacks occur, do not be discouraged. Remember that losing weight and weight maintenance are part of life and part of your lifestyle.

Failures and Disappointments

Your life and the world around you are filled with many obstacles and problems. Everyone fails at one time or another. It is part of life, and it is inevitable. We feel sad when we fail. Failure is looked on by society as a defeat. The higher the standard you set for yourself, the harder and more bitter the failures will seem.

Failures can also bring not only a feeling of disappointment but also sadness. Disappointment means falling short of achieving one's goals. Therefore, when you set a goal for yourself, make sure it is realistic and achievable. Think of a major goal as many smaller and achievable goals! Celebrate each accomplishment—no matter how small—and set a new goal right away. After any failure or disappointment, it is important that you examine the situation and the goal thoroughly. In addition, you should also ask yourself, "What were the reasons for this failure?" "What can I do to avoid it next time?" "Was the set goal a realistic goal?" "How should I approach it next time?" Most failures don't prove a lack of ability; they generally reflect a lack of conviction.

You may also underestimate your powers and abilities. Most self-limits have never been tested or challenged by you. You have a misconception about your limits, because you have not pushed yourself to the limit. Do you really believe that the top athletes or performers of great feats were able to do these extreme tasks without numerous trials and failures? Self-handicapping is the worst behavior. You have set your mind and body for failure before you have even tried.

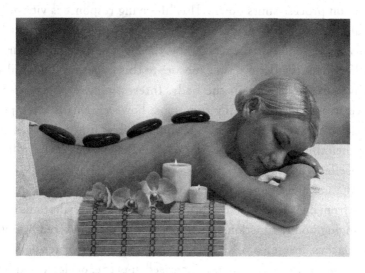

VIII. Thou Shalt Reduce Your Stress

Stress is any reaction to a stimulus that impairs the stability and balance of the body's physiological functions. Physical, mental, and emotional factors can work in concert to make you stressed and ultimately overweight. Physical and chemical factors that can cause stress include trauma, infections, toxins, illnesses, and injuries. Emotional causes of stress are plentiful and varied as well.

If stress disrupts the body's balance and function, are all levels of stress bad for you? The answer is a simple no. Some level of stress is good for you. Stress is often thought of in a negative light, and with good reason. However, stress, both physical and emotional, also helps your body stay active, alert, and more prepared for obstacles it may face. So, low levels of stress and tension can occasionally be beneficial. This is the famous fight-or-flight response. The response of our body to any stress is reflected in the reaction of our nervous system. When we are faced with either real or imaginary danger, our minds prepare our body to carry out one of these two conditions: fight or flight. The manifestation of preparedness is in the form of increased heart rate, higher blood pressure, and the temporary shutting down of unnecessary bodily functions, such as digestion and defecation. Breathing becomes shallow, muscles tense in anticipation of action, and blood flow to vital organs is decreased. The digestive and elimination process shuts down. This lifesaving response is vital for our survival, as our body is prepared to defend itself. However, if our body remains in this condition for a long time, the flight or fight can be harmful. It is self-evident that long-term exposure to this hyperphysiological state will have adverse effects on the body. Interestingly, even exercise can produce stress on some bodily functions; however, this is a temporary response, and the health benefits are indisputable. It is only when stress is overwhelming and continuous, or poorly managed, that its harmful and negative effects appear.

Symptoms and signs of excessive or poorly controlled stress can vary in extreme from one individual to another. These signs and symptoms include wide-ranging bodily functions. You may suffer stress-induced symptoms like headaches, insomnia or sleep disturbances, anxiety or tension, anger, lack of concentration, depression, increased appetite, or decreased libido. If left unattended, these can lead to severe and overwhelming stress, to the point of so-called burnout. Burnout is the point at which there is a loss of interest in all type of normal activities. One should avoid reaching this point if possible. Stress can ultimately affect your immune system and any underlying medical conditions. Stress releases corticosteroids, which are rapidly converted to cortisol in the bloodstream, and elevated levels of these have an immunosuppressive effect. If you are stressed, you are more susceptible to catching colds, infections, and illnesses.

Stress Hormones

Two adrenal hormones, DHEA (dehydroepiandrosterone) and cortisol, are your body's main forces for coping with stress. The balance of these two hormones can affect how you handle the overwhelming feelings that stress can bring.

When your body feels stress, cortisol is essential. Cortisol adjusts your energy levels to assist your body during that stressful period. DHEA is the most abundant androgen—male— steroid, and is secreted by the adrenal glands and, to a lesser extent, by the ovaries and testes. DHEA can be converted into other steroid hormones, including testosterone and estrogen. In addition, DHEA may play a role in the aging process. Together, DHEA and cortisol work to provide your body with an optimal stress response.

DHEA and cortisol are released into your bloodstream from your adrenal glands when your body feels stress and help your body make the necessary adjustments to protect it. These two hormones help balance each other to ensure a stress response.

DHEA is an anabolic hormone, a hormone that affects the immune system, blood pressure, and sleep, among its many other functions. Anabolic steroids are a class of steroidal hormones related to the hormone testosterone. They increase protein synthesis within cells, which results in the buildup of cellular tissue (anabolism), especially in muscles. Furthermore, anabolic steroids also have androgenic and virilizing properties, including the development and maintenance of masculine characteristics, such as the thickening of the vocal cords and growth of body hair.

Cortisol is a catabolic hormone, a hormone that also affects the immune system, blood pressure, and sleep. Catabolic steroids, like natural hydrocortisone, help the body break down tissues to release glucose—sugar—and mobilize energy in response to stress or danger.

Comparing your levels of DHEA and cortisol to the general population will help to establish a benchmark for comparison. With this information, you can work with your family physician to develop an appropriate program to maintain and promote your good health.

Cortisol and Eating

Cortisol levels in your blood can build up during long-term stress situations. This buildup can make you feel hungry, even when you're not—especially for carbohydrate-rich and high-sugar foods. Cortisol can even elevate blood pressure and heart rate.

When you are under stress, your body gives you an adrenalin rush, the fight-or-flight response discussed earlier. Considering the way society is structured, it is unlikely that you will be able to accomplish the appropriate fight-or-flight response when it is called for whenever everyday stress occurs. Instead, you tend to suppress your natural response, which is driven by hormones that are, quite simply, not suppressed.

Interestingly, comfort eating when you are stressed is one of the main reasons your waistline expands.

Comfort Eating and Weight Gain

As human beings, our eating patterns are regulated not just by whether we are hungry but also by social cues in the environment. You eat dinner or lunch because it's the proper time for eating, or because your family or friends want to have a meal. Eating behavior and eating disorders are very complex, with environmental, emotional, physical, nutritional, and social components. Comfort eating is mostly psychological. The reason some people continue to eat even when they are not hungry is to comfort their feelings of stress, depression, and anger; they want and need to be loved. What you need to do is find something to substitute for eating to calm your nerves. In some cases, the eating comes from more than everyday stress. In that case, you might need to talk to a professional about the problems.

Food Addiction

Overweight and obesity are on the rise in the United States. The numbers are growing at an alarming rate. During the past twenty years, there has been a dramatic increase in obesity in the United States. Currently, more than 64 percent of US adults are either overweight or obese, according to results from the 1999–2000 National Health and Nutrition Examination Survey (NHANES IV). This figure represents a 14 percent increase from NHANES III (1988–94), and a 36 percent increase from NHANES II (1976–80). The greatest increase took place in the obese group (BMI > 30), where the prevalence doubled from NHANES II. Roughly fifty-nine million American adults are in the obese group, which is at the greatest health risk.

Compulsive behavior and disturbed sleep patterns are two of the major signs of addiction. The important aspect of addictive behaviors is that the time between the craving and the reinforcement is immediate. That's why fast foods are so effective. Are the high-fat, sugar-laden things we crave addictive?

It has been shown that parts of the brain of an overeater have a lesser amount of dopamine, a neurotransmitter associated with motivation and pleasure, receptors than the brain of someone with normal eating habits (85–88). This is also true in the case of drug addicts, who have a similar shortage of dopamine receptors. This is your brain on drugs.

Interestingly, it has also been verified that the mere sight and smell of food can release dopamine (89, 90). So, can food have a role similar to narcotics? To compensate for low dopamine, overeaters have to consume more food to get the same response experienced by individuals with normal levels of dopamine. This may be the same reason drug addicts use narcotics. These facts alone cannot explain overeating. But eating is tied in with comfort and caring.

Can Stress Make You Overweight?

Yes! Stress and weight are closely related. Discharges of your hormones are not only under the influence of your emotions and physical conditions, your emotions can be influenced and manipulated by the hormones that ultimately affect your eating habits. The hormone adrenaline, for example, is released to help you deal with stress. Adrenaline is released whenever we are excited, frightened, or anxious. This will speed up your metabolic rate and ultimately, promote weight loss. On the other hand, long-term and poorly controlled stress can have a harmful and negative effect. As discussed previously, cortisol, also released when you are stressed, can increase fat storage, predominantly in the abdominal area. In other words, short-lived stress may help us to lose weight, but long-term stress can make us gain weight.

Cortisol is one of the chief hormones released when you are feeling stressed. High levels of cortisol in your bloodstream reduces protein in most body cells. It also signals the body to eat more carbohydrate-rich foods and store them as fat. The bottom line is that ongoing stress can cause cortisol obesity. You are well aware of binge eating during stressful times. Comfort eating during stressful moments—which tend to be many—often causes one's waistline to increase and fitness to decrease. In addition, high levels of cortisol are directly associated with elevated blood sugar level, diabetes, and accelerated hair and bone loss. Long-term high levels of cortisol are also linked to reduced states of immunity and increased risk of infections.

Suppress Cortisol

Cortisol is responsible for triggering the breakdown of protein (such as muscle tissue) into building blocks called amino acids. It also inhibits glucose from getting into the cells, causing a further wasting of muscle. Cortisol is also a "junk food" hormone: high levels of cortisol generally trigger a strong craving for high-carbohydrate snacks. Several things raise your cortisol level: lack of food, lack of sleep, prolonged high-intensity or high-impact exercise, and weight lifting. This is why your workouts should generally not exceed about an hour. Bottom line: several forms of stress trigger cortisol, and your job is to shut it down.

Cortisol can elevate your blood pressure and your heart rate. It is well known that avoiding stress is nearly impossible in our fast-paced life. Therefore, it is best to attempt to decrease the body's release of cortisol (see table 1). Moderate exercise and lovemaking, along with sufficient sleep and a healthy low-calorie diet, can significantly lower cortisol levels. Some dietary supplements can help, including a multivitamin, vitamin C, and folic acid. Furthermore, avoid too much caffeine, nicotine, and alcohol, because they can create cycles of stress and fatigue.

Table 1: Activities to Reduce Stress

+ Aromatherapy
+ Bathing (bubble bath)
+ Dancing
+ Deep breathing
+ Drink water
+ Eat light healthy and unprocessed foods for snacks, such as fruits, vegetables, and yogurt
+ Gardening
+ Hugging
+ Kissing Laughter

- Light physical activities
- Lovemaking
- Massage therapy
- Music
- Painting
- Physical rest
- Playing an instrument
- Playing with your pet
- Praying
- Reading
- Showering
- Singing
- Sleep
- Stretching
- Swimming
- Talking with a friend
- Walking
- Yoga

Massage and Weight Loss

To achieve physical fitness, you can take advantage of massage therapy. Some of the major benefits of massage therapy are increased blood flow, improved circulation, reduced stress and the elimination of tension, reduced muscle aches and stiffness, and improved muscle and joint function. Massage also increases your body's self-awareness and sensitivity; reduces anxiety levels; relaxes, focuses, and clears your mind; fulfills your need for a nurturing touch and intimacy; improves self-esteem: and instills a general sense of well-being. Last but not least, it feels good.

Massage can reveal the caring and loving feelings of couples and improve their level of intimacy. By giving massages, one can also burn calories: it is a physical activity. So, give love, and in return, be pampered. Use aromatherapy to enhance your experience and the pleasure.

Aromatherapy

As far back as the dawn of history, herbal medicine, using pure, essential plant extracts, has been in use. Research has shown that certain aromas do produce distinct physical effects (91–102). Scents of certain essential oils stimulate the production of serotonin, while others relax you and ease your pain. Serotonin is produced in the brain and has many properties, including a sedative effect. For example, scents of commonly used and available condiments and food additives—such as vanilla, orange blossom, rose, chamomile, and lavender—have a calming effect, while sandalwood, lavender, eucalyptus, and nutmeg help you resist negative effects of stress. Some herbal therapies are used for several divergent properties. For example, lavender can not only help you to relax and fight stress, it also eases aches and pains, such as headaches.

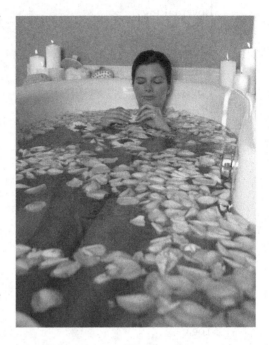

Sexual Aromatherapy and Scents as Aphrodisiacs

We are affected by all the scents around us, including the scents of others, especially those of of our lover. By adorning yourself with certain scents or adding the right scents to your bedroom and home, you can create a sensual and romantic atmosphere your lover is sure to respond to. Hence, scent can be considered the silent language of sexuality and sensuality.

Remarkably, the sense of smell is directly linked to the part of the brain related to memory and emotion. Research studies have shown that different scents can actually produce different emotions and reactions. Moreover, aromas can affect the human subconscious and cause physiological reactions, such as changes in the level of blood pressure, rate of respiration, and heartbeat, which are mainly under involuntary control. You are not aware of the fact that you have to breathe and your heart has to pump. These physiological processes are basically under sympathetic control.

Our sense of smell is approximately ten thousand times more sensitive than our sense of taste. For example, a healthy young person can distinguish and recognize over thousands of different odors. No wonder—once a smell is encountered it is rarely forgotten. A familiar scent can stir basic emotions, and distant memories can be recalled instantly—just from the hint of a familiar scent.

How Does Aromatherapy Work?

All the essential oils used in aromatherapy have their own unique aroma and pharmacological effect on your body. Aromatherapy, like any other fragrance, directly stimulates the brain via the olfactory nerves, which provide the sense of smell, in your nasal passages. The area of the brain associated with the sense of smell is called the olfactory system which consists of the olfactory bulb, the olfactory nerve, and the mucous membranes. The olfactory bulb is the main part which transmits information to the brain. This is also the most direct contact our brain has with its immediate environment—the essential oils, aromas, etc. Since the olfactory system is very closely connected to the limbic system—the area of the brain which is said to contain our most basic drives, such as thirst, hunger, and sex drive. In addition, this limbic system also modulates our most subtle responses such as our emotions, memories, creativity, and intuition.

Furthermore, The olfactory system also connects to the hypothalamus and pituitary glands. The hypothalamus controls our primitive emotions, such as fear, pleasure, rage, lust, and bliss, while the pituitary is the master gland which governs all other glands in the body as well as controlling the autonomic nervous system. These nerves stimulate the limbic system in the brain that influences emotions and memories. This effect is so strong that a simple scent can bring back lovely memories of your childhood. Amazingly, the effect on the limbic system can be directly linked to the adrenals, pituitary gland, and the hypothalamus—the parts of the body that regulate heart rate, blood pressure, stress, memory, hormone balance, and breathing.

It is important to mention that due to the unique molecular structure and characteristic of these volatile oils, scents, and aromas, their physiologic and psychological effect on the human physiology and psyche is very rapid and brisk since they directly affect the limbic system and the brain as a whole. Simply put, the direct stimulation of the olfactory bulb in the nasal and sinuses immediately affects the brain! Emotional and physiological effects are so immediate, aromatherapy can be compared to an intravenous form of drug therapy!

Aromatherapy and Weight Loss

Have you ever cooked a dish or sauce with a fantastic and mouth-watering smell on the stovetop or the grill? If you can recall, you will recognize that when you sat down to eat the dish, you were not hungry anymore—or not as hungry as you had thought.

In addition to the effect of scent and smell on your limbic system, aroma and scents can affect the satiety centers in your brain. The satiety centers inform you when you are full and satisfied. These centers directly activate your olfactory system. As mentioned before, your nose and the olfactory nerves are the only sensing system in your body with direct input to the brain, making smell a highly sensitive and important sense. There are certain aromas that stimulate the appetite and ones that suppress the appetite.

Any food aroma that you enjoy will stimulate your appetite; however, the expectations and time of day are influences too. Popular appetizing food aromas include baking bread, garlic, and chocolate chip cookies. However, these food aromas will only stimulate your appetite when you are hungry. Interestingly, any of these aromas would not have a major effect on your appetite if you'd just eaten your fill. On the other hand, some essential oils (fennel, bergamot, cardamom, and so on), and foods containing them, have reputation for curbing the appetite. Fennel can help with weight control and improved digestion. Smelling fennel essential oil can also work to help control appetite. It should be emphasized that people may have a different reaction to some of the aromas. Therefore, everyone should keep a mental log of the aromas that have a special effect on their appetite.

Aromatherapy employs the essential oils extracted from aromatic plants to elicit a positive, healthy response. These essential oils can relax and soothe the mind and body, as well as energize and invigorate the spirit.

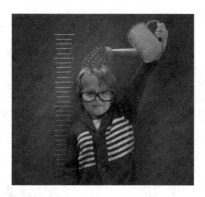

IX. Thou Shalt Nourish Your Mind

Several research studies over the past several decades have confirmed the strong link between the body and the mind. In a landmark study published in 1991 in the *Journal of the American Medical Association*, it was found that pregnant women who were assisted by a trained support person during childbirth had greatly reduced rates of caesarean section and anesthesia use (103, 104). A clinical study conducted by Italian researchers, which was published in the *Journal of Rheumatology*, involved more than sixty patients suffering from osteoarthritis of the knee. It was found that the level of depression better predicted the patients' disabilities and pain than did the extent of their knee damage. In a study of approximately two hundred patients with heart disease, researchers at the University of Washington found that measures of anxiety and depression better predicted patients' health status one year after cardiac catheterization than did the severity of narrowing in the coronary arteries. In a Duke University study of 107 patients with heart disease, researchers found that relaxation, cognitive therapy, and a lowering of hostility reduced the risk of further heart problems by 75 percent, compared to patients given the usual medical care and medications. Interestingly, in a larger study at UC Davis, 335 patients about to undergo surgery were randomly assigned to listen to one of four different audiotapes before and after surgery. The group that listened to a tape with guided imagery, music, and specific suggestions of diminished blood loss and rapid healing had 43 percent less blood loss and spent one less day in the hospital, compared to people who listened to other kinds of tapes (105–109).

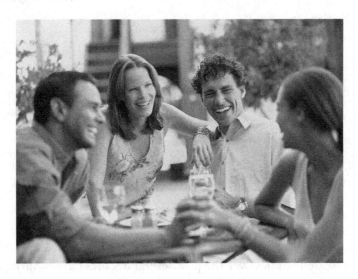

Laughter and Health

In many studies, laughter has been found to lower blood pressure, reduce stress hormones, and boost immune function (110–119). Laughter also initiates the release of endorphins, natural painkillers produced by your brain, which give you a general sense of well-being.

It is clinically proven that laughter is a wonderful stress-reducer and a great mood-lifter (116–119). It also lowers serum cortisol levels and stimulates the immune system; this counteracts the immunosuppressive effects of stress. Your emotional experiences directly affect your immune system. A sense of humor allows us to perceive and appreciate the tough and stressful incidents of life and provides moments of joy and delight. These positive emotions can create neurochemical changes that buffer the immunosuppressive effects of stress.

Laughter causes muscle relaxation, reduces stress hormones, enhances your immune system, reduces pain, and reduces blood pressure. So laugh; it is good.

Your Mood Affects How You Look!

It is a fact that when you are down or not in a good mood, you do not look your best. Your mood and inner thoughts can radiate through you externally. You look better and more confident when you are in a good mood.

When you are in a bad mood, it shows, and it can affect others' interactions with you. Just ask them. It is like listening to a sad song or looking at a sad picture. You can alienate friends, relatives, coworkers. Of course, life can hand you lemons and put you in a bad mood. Even in these down and blue times, a positive attitude and looking on the bright side can help.

So, look to enhance your beauty. Every person is born with certain beauty. Look for it and enhance it. Forget about the anorexic and severely emaciated looks that Hollywood—more accurately called "Hollow wood"—represents.

Take good care of yourself inside and out. Groom yourself, do your hair, dress nice, and, ladies, put on makeup. Put on your good perfume/cologne, and start loving yourself. And start the L.O.V.E. diet.

Singing and Weight Loss

If you like to sing, try it when you feel low and blue. Turn up your favorite song, and sing it at the top of your lungs. There's something about singing that's almost utterly opposed to feeling down. Of course, you should sing an upbeat tune rather than the blues. Singing one song tends to burn between ten and twenty kilocalories. Naturally, the longer and livelier the singing, the more calories you burn. So, go on and sing with all your might. In the shower, in your car, anywhere you can. Turn on your favorite music and sing along, and move with the music. Roll up the car windows and sing loudly. Bottom line, sing anywhere you can and as loudly as you can. Sing yourself into a better mood.

Listen to feel-good music the next time you have the urge to binge. Researchers have discovered that uplifting music can activate the same "feel-good" center in your brain, just as eating your favorite foods does.

Physical Benefits of Touching

Do you remember the strong embrace of a friend in times of difficulty or a hug from your mom when you didn't feel well?

We are living things who need and require human touch and contact for growth and well-being. Hugging can be sexual and nonsexual. Overall, a good hug can warm your relationships. Hugs make you feel good. A hug is a natural and easy way to tell someone that you care. Like touch, it can be life-giving and healing. Touching helps alleviate the pain and anguish. The need for touch and hugs exists in us at birth, and we don't lose the desire or need for touch as we grow.

We humans, being social beings, need more than just good nutrition and good physical care. There is an inherent need for physical contact, including hugs. The quote, "A hug is a special gift: it can always be returned, and one size fits all," says it all. Hugging is a way of showing your genuine affection and appreciation, and it is also a means of connecting with people you care about. It can say things for which you don't have words. The nicest thing about a hug is that you usually can't give one without getting one. A hug makes you feel good.

When at a loss for words, one simple sincere hug can transfer all your concern, care, and well wishes. Sometimes, a good hug from someone you care about can make all the difference. So hug your friends, your coworkers, your spouse, your children, your relatives.

The physical and emotional effects of hugging are many. Hugging and touching, which are different forms of physical contact, have physical and emotional effects on the giver and the receiver. A hug can make a difference in a person's state of mind and physical ailment. Therefore, hugging is good medicine. Hugging is natural and possibly an innate movement that is ingrained in us for survival. We are "hardwired" to thrive as social beings.

Hugging is good medicine. It transfers energy and gives the person hugged an emotional boost. Hugs are not only nice, they are needed. Hugs can relieve pain and depression. They make the healthier happier, and the most secure even more so. Hugging feels good and overcomes fear. It provides a stretching exercise for short people and a stooping exercise for tall people. Hugging does not upset the environment. It saves heat and energy and requires no special equipment. Hugging makes happy days happier and impossible days possible.

Touch can lower production of cortisol, a stress hormone. When our cortisol level drops, there is an increase in production of two brain chemicals: serotonin and dopamine. These chemicals in our brain are responsible for the state of euphoria, making us feel good.

Even though we are much more physical and "touchy-feely" in public compared to most Asian cultures, compared to French couples, we are way behind.

Scientific investigations into the effects of touch support the theory that stimulation by touch is utterly necessary for our physical as well as our emotional well-being (120–127). Therapeutic touch has been recognized as a vital tool for caring and expediting healing in nursing and medicine. No wonder it has become the cornerstone of education in many nursing and medical schools. The sense of touch can be manipulated to relieve and or reduce pains and aches, decrease depression, alleviate anxiety, and bring out a sense of well-being and a will to live. A variety of experiments have shown that touch can have a positive effect on an infant's development, growth, and IQ. Scientists are just beginning to discover and unravel the enormous powers of physical touch and hugging. It has been shown that these forms of physical interaction can ease your tension, relax you, make you feel good about yourself, fight off insomnia, impart feelings of belonging and caring, and reduce your overall stress.

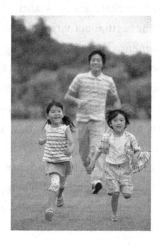

X. Thou Shalt Increase Your Physical Activity

You might be too busy to go to the fitness club or gym on a regular basis. Like most people, you probably lack the motivation for a scheduled and strict exercise regimen. However, physical activity need not be performed in a gym! Remember, any physical activity is a form of exercise.

Physical Activity and Health

There is plenty of scientific evidence to support the fact that people who lead active lifestyles are less likely to suffer from major illnesses, such as heart disease, diabetes, and colon cancer. In addition, increased physical activity is linked to longevity and better health. Regular exercise can increase levels of HDL (good cholesterol), lower blood pressure, improve body composition, lower blood-sugar levels, improve bone density, boost the immune system, improve mood, and reduce chances of depression.

Despite the overwhelming evidence for regular exercise, many people do not do regular exercises. This is due to several reasons: lack of time, cost of equipment or fitness club membership, and lack of stamina and stress. The biggest difficulty is the inability to incorporate physical activity in their lives due to many other commitments. One of the reasons people allow these obstacles to get in their way is that they believe only vigorous exercise counts. So, if they can't do something strenuous, they don't do anything at all.

It is a myth that only vigorous exercise or playing sports count as healthy activity. The good news is that there are substantial health benefits that can be attained from many of the regular activities of daily living. These activities don't require special equipment. There is now strong scientific evidence that moderate intensity physical activity—equivalent to brisk walking for thirty minutes per day on most days of the week—is enough to bring about real benefits in terms of promoting health and preventing illnesses (128).

Regular activity can also improve the way you look and feel. In combination with a balanced diet, regular activity can help to maintain a healthy weight. It can even boost self-confidence and reduce the risk of depression. If you decide to start exercising, it's important to start gently, increasing the frequency of your activity gradually, and later increasing the intensity level of the exercise. This is especially important if you have been sedentary or are very out of shape.

How Much Physical Activity Is Enough?

Moderate physical activity is one of thirty minutes' duration. During moderate-intensity activity, you should be able to talk without panting.

During a moderate-intensity physical activity, you can burn up to two hundred calories. You can accomplish these thirty minutes of physical activity in three ten-minute sessions.

You can achieve your daily target fairly simply. Examples of everyday activities that count include using the stairs instead of taking the elevator, dancing, walking, gardening, and parking at the end of the lot when shopping.

To keep up with your physical activity plan, find an activity or activities that you enjoy. If you find a particular physical activity boring, it will be very difficult to sustain. Try new activities until you find one that you like. Try to get your friends or family involved, so you can motivate each other. Remember, many common activities, such as singing, dancing, and walking, can help you burn calories.

Set yourself some short- and long-term goals. Success will provide you with a sense of satisfaction. Make sure to reward yourself every time you achieve your goals, and try to incorporate those activities into your regular daily routine.

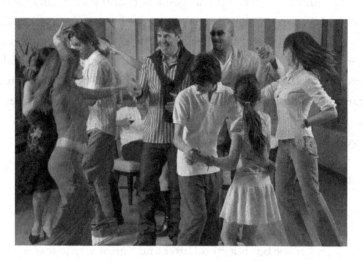

Dancing and Weight Loss

Dancing is a great way to help your body drop a few unwanted pounds. It's also a fun way to exercise. Many athletes incorporate dance workouts into their fitness programs for better balance, alignment, and flexibility.

Dancing is a great form of exercise. You may find exercises boring, as many people do, but you can dance off your excess calories. Most forms of dancing are aerobic in nature, therefore, you burn fat and tone your muscles. One hour of dancing can burn, on average, three hundred to four hundred calories.

All forms of dancing burn calories, because dance involves movement, and energy is required for every movement made. The calorie-burning ability of each dance depends on the speed or force at which it is performed.

The more vigorous the exercise, the more calories you burn. For example, with one hour of ballroom dancing, you burn about two hundred calories; with rock and roll or salsa, you burn about four hundred calories; and with country dancing, you burn approximately three hundred calories.

This estimation of calories burned is based on a 150-pound person. The heavier you are, the more calories you will burn, and vice versa.

Dancing Improves Fitness

Most aerobic exercise helps your body to burn fat if maintained for more than twenty minutes. Dancing is as good as running and other moderate exercises and is an optimal way to improve your fitness. You can reach your desired heart rate (60 to 85 percent of your estimated maximum heart rate) through many forms of dance. From burning calories to socializing with friends, dancing of any kind offers these health benefits: it improves your cardiovascular conditioning, makes your bones stronger, tones your muscles, improves your flexibility, makes your heart stronger, makes your lungs work better, and ultimately, improves your self-esteem.

Belly Dancing

One of the most fun exercises around is belly dancing. Belly dancing is both an art and an exercise. Belly dancing dates back two thousand years. It is not only exotic and erotic but is a mood lifter and a great way to lose unwanted weight. As with all forms of physical activity, the number of calories burned during belly dancing depends on the intensity of the dance. There are also different levels of dancing. On average, you can lose three hundred to four hundred calories with an intense one-hour session. There are many other benefits to belly dancing: you can tone your muscles, trim the lower body (hips, waist, legs), and boost your romantic life.

Belly dancing is considered a great cardio workout that can strengthen muscles through isolation movements. It is low impact, but it will certainly make you sweat.

Great News!

Lovemaking can help you develop a trim body, shiny skin, healthy blood, a healthy heart, and healthy bones. In brief, you can "sex-ercise" to lose weight, feel great, and get into shape!

Table 2. Activities to Substitute for Exercise

Belly dance	Bathe
Canoe	Bicycle
Chew	Carry your own groceries
Cook	Clean
Fish	Dance
Hike	Garden
Kiss	Hug
Paint	Make love
Play ball	Row
Sauna	Shop
Shower	Sing
Swim	Walk
Take the stairs	Window shop

Chapter Two

Basic Nutrition: Facts and Tools

In this chapter, I review the basic terminology and concepts in nutrition. You can use this chapter as a quick reference when planning daily or weekly menus and as a guide to what you should know when attempting to eat healthy.

Major Nutrients in the Diet

Nutrients are usually divided into five major classes:

1. Carbohydrates

2. Proteins

3. Fats (oils)

4. Vitamins

5. Minerals

Proteins, carbohydrates, and fats/oils are usually called macronutrients. Vitamins and minerals are usually called micronutrients.

The Glycemic Index

The glycemic index (Glycemic Index) was developed in 1980 to assist diabetics in better controlling their blood-sugar levels and avoiding dangerous increases in blood sugar. It is a gauge of how fast a food is digested and absorbed into the gastrointestinal tract. This characteristic has a direct effect on your blood-sugar levels. Low-Glycemic Index foods increase energy levels throughout the day. The higher the Glycemic Index of any food, the faster its digestion and absorption and the faster the rise in blood-glucose level. This means there is an immediate rush of energy, but it is shortlived.

After the initial burst of energy after consuming high-Glycemic Index foods, the resulting insulin response removes the sugar from your blood, and you begin to feel fatigued. Eating foods low on the Glycemic Index will keep you from going through this roller coaster of high and low blood sugar. Your blood-sugar levels will remain more level throughout the day, which will give you a feeling of high energy all day long. Low-Glycemic Index carbohydrates will also help nondiabetics with weight reduction.

The Glycemic Index of a specific food can vary. Cooking, especially overcooking foods, will increase their Glycemic Index. The Glycemic Index of bananas will increase as they ripen. The Glycemic Index of pasta can vary by protein content, size, and even shape.

Basically foods are divided into three major categories:

1. High-Glycemic Index Foods—80 or above
   Examples: glucose, honey, candies, cookies, jelly beans, sports drinks, bagels, wheat cereals, white rice, baked potatoes, watermelon, fruit juices, white breads, white rice, croissants, corn flakes, candy, drinks, beer, and alcohol.

2. Medium-Glycemic Index Foods—40–80
   Examples: Breakfast bar, tortilla chips, whole-wheat breads, brown rice, boiled potatoes, and bananas.

3. Low-Glycemic Index Foods–40 or below

Therefore, attempt to eat more of the following foods that have low Glycemic Index numbers as well as contain high fiber. Simply think "unprocessed." Carbohydrates that are refined and have had most if not all of the fiber removed are digested much more rapidly and cause a rise in blood-sugar level. Good choices include, milk, pasta, bran cereals, beans, chocolate, sponge cakes, apples, oranges, pears, bananas, other fresh fruits, oatmeal, brown rice, whole-wheat pasta, barley, basmati rice, whole grains, peas, lentils, corn, potato with skin, yams, yogurt, and soy.

Proteins

Proteins are essential nutrients required by your body to maintain your health at an optimal level. Proteins are made up of a long chain of amino acids connected together linearly. Your body uses these amino acids—building blocks—to create new proteins to repair, replace, and heal the damaged tissues in your body. Proteins can also function in other ways, such as play an important part of molecule to transport oxygen and nutrients in your blood and cells, regulate growth, act as hormones, regulate electrolytes and water balance, create antibodies to fight infections, and maintain the integrity of cells, tissues, and vital organs.

You need approximately 0.3 to 0.4 grams of protein per pound of body weight per day. Plant proteins are superior to animal protein. Clinical evidence shows that people who are on a vegetarian diet are generally healthier and live longer than nonvegetarians counterparts. They have lower rates of coronary disease, hypertension, type II diabetes, obesity, osteoporosis, dementia, and many types of cancers (129–133). Vegetarian diets tend to be rich in complex carbohydrates, omega-6 fatty acids, dietary fiber, carotenoids, folic acid, vitamin C, vitamin E, potassium, and magnesium. In addition, they are generally low in saturated fat and cholesterol (132, 133).

The following is a short list of different food categories with adequate content of protein.

+ Nuts: hazelnuts, Brazil nuts, almonds, cashews, walnuts, pine nuts
+ Seeds: sesame, pumpkin, sunflower
+ Legumes: peas, beans, lentils, peanuts
+ Grains/cereals: wheat, all types of high-fiber flour, pasta, barley, rye, oats, corn, rice
+ Soy products: tofu, vegetable protein, veggie burgers, and soymilk
+ Dairy products: milk, cheese, and yogurt
+ Eggs
+ Meat, poultry, fish, seafood

Carbohydrates

Carbohydrates (sugars) are divided into three main types:

1. Simple sugars (high-Glycemic Index carbohydrates)

2. Complex sugars or starches (low-Glycemic Index carbohydrates)

3. Dietary fiber (indigestible complex sugars)

Simple sugars can be found in fruit juices, milk, and ordinary sugar.

Complex sugars are found in cereals, grains, bread, rice, pasta, oats, barley, rye, whole fruits, and vegetables, such as potatoes and parsnips. Unrefined carbohydrates, like whole-wheat bread and brown rice, are best, because they contain essential dietary fiber.

Fiber

Fiber is a carbohydrate subgroup. There are two types of fiber: soluble and insoluble. Insoluble fiber is found in cereals such as wheat bran and fibrous fruit and vegetables. It absorbs water, thus making you feel fuller, and helps to slow down the absorption of simple sugars from the gut into the bloodstream, thus averting hypoglycemia and improving the passage of undigested material through the bowel, preventing constipation, and helping to rid the body of toxins. Soluble fiber is to be found in many fruits, vegetables, and oat bran. It can be transported in the bloodstream, where it binds with fat and helps to prevent atherosclerosis.

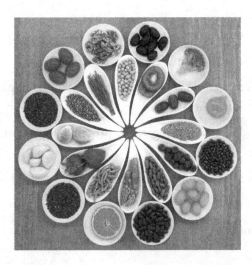

Unless your diet is high in fiber, you run the risk of other serious diseases, including bowel cancer, coronary disease, diabetes, and gallstones. These diseases may not be related to fiber content alone but may be influenced by levels of carbohydrates, protein, and animal fat as well.

Dietary Fiber Functions and Benefits (427)

Functions	Benefits
Adds bulk to your diet, making you feel full faster	May reduce appetite
Attracts water and turns to gel during digestion, trapping carbohydrates and slowing absorption of glucose	Lowers variance in blood sugar levels
Lowers total and LDL cholesterol	Reduces risk of heart disease
Regulates blood sugar	Reduces onset risk or symptoms of metabolic syndrome and diabetes
Speeds the passage of foods through the digestive system	Facilitates regularity
Adds bulk to the stool	Alleviates constipation
Balances intestinal pH	Stimulates intestinal fermentation production of short-chain
Reduces risk of colorectal cancer	fatty acids

Adapted from http://en.wikipedia.org/wiki/Dietary_fiber.

Dietary Fiber

Regular consumption of a diet rich in fiber has many potential health benefits. These include reduced risk of stroke, heart disease, and adult-onset diabetes (DM type II; 207–208). In addition, a high intake of dietary fiber is commonly recommended as treatment for digestive irregularities like constipation, diarrhea, and hemorrhoids. Dietary fiber is commonly found in legumes (beans, lentils, and peas), grains, vegetables, and fruits. However, most Americans do not consume enough fiber as is commonly recommended.

It is important to emphasize that there is no single dietary fiber. In the past, fiber was considered to be only that substance found in the outer layers of grains or plants (like the outer layer of wheat grain, called wheat bran), which was believed to be indigestible by the human digestive system. That simplistic and partly erroneous notion has changed, and we now know that fiber actually consists of a number of different substances. Therefore, the term "dietary fiber" should be used, which includes many different substances. Since most dietary fiber is not digested or absorbed by the human digestive system, it stays within the intestine, where it aids in the digestion of other foods and affects the consistency of stool.

Dietary fiber consists of two types of fiber, each with its own health benefits:

1. Soluble fiber

2. Insoluble fiber

Soluble fiber consists of a group of substances that is made of carbohydrates and dissolves in water. Examples of foods that contain soluble fiber include fruits, oats, barley, and legumes like lentils, peas, and beans.

Insoluble fiber is derived from the walls of plant cells and does not dissolve in water. Examples of foods that contain insoluble fiber include wheat, rye, and other common grains. The commonly used wheat bran is a type of insoluble fiber.

Benefits of a High-Fiber Diet

The differences between health benefits of these two types of fiber are not very clear. However, there are several potential benefits of eating a diet rich in dietary fiber. For example, insoluble fiber (wheat bran and some fruits and vegetables) has been recommended to treat digestive problems, such as constipation, hemorrhoids, chronic diarrhea, and fecal incontinence. Fiber bulks and softens the stool and, thereby, makes bowel movements easier and more regular.

As for the soluble fiber (psyllium, pectin, wheat dextrin, and other products), they can reduce the risk of coronary artery disease and stroke by approximately 50 percent compared to a low-fiber diet (134–138). In addition, soluble fiber can reduce the risk of developing adult onset diabetes. Moreover, in diabetics (types 1 and 2), soluble fiber can help to control blood-glucose levels, as it avoids surge in blood sugar by slowing and regulating its absorption.

The recommended daily intake of dietary fiber is twenty-five grams for women and thirty grams for men (134–138). Dietary sources of fiber include:

+ Fruits
+ Vegetables

+ Cereals

+ Fiber supplements (psyllium, methylcellulose, and calcium polycarbophil)

Adding fiber to the diet can have some side effects, such as abdominal bloating or gas. To minimize these side effects, consumption of dietary fiber and fiber supplement should be started with a small amount and increased slowly, until stools become softer and more frequent. And since the fiber in the supplements is mostly soluble, it should be taken with plenty of water. Keep in mind that some people, including those with irritable bowel syndrome, do better by not increasing fiber in their diet (138–141).

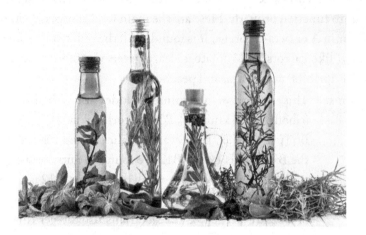

Fats and Oils

Fats can be divided into two major types:

1. Saturated

2. Unsaturated

   + Monounsaturated

   + Polyunsaturated

Fats are made of smaller units called fatty acids. Two of these fatty acids, linoleic and linolenic acids, are essential fatty acids (EFAs), as they must be provided in the diet for proper cell metabolism and physiology. EFAs are necessary fats that humans cannot synthesize and that cannot be assembled within the body from other components by any known chemical pathways; therefore, they must be obtained through diet. The term refers to fatty acids involved in vital and important biological processes for a healthy body, and not those that just play a role as fuel. EFAs are long-chain polyunsaturated fatty acids derived from linolenic, linoleic, and oleic acids. Plant foods are rich in EFAs. Vegetable fats are mainly the unsaturated type. Animal fats have a tendency to be more saturated.

Vitamins

Vitamins are a group of heterogeneous and unrelated nutrients that your body cannot synthesize. Your body needs only very small quantities of vitamins to function properly. Here are the main food sources of vitamins:

Vitamin A or beta-carotene: It is found in all the red, orange, or yellow vegetables like carrots and tomatoes, leafy green vegetables and certain fruits like apricots, nectarines, and peaches.

B vitamins: This group of vitamins includes B1 (thiamin), B2 (riboflavin), B3 (niacin), B5 (pantothenic acid), B7 (biotin), B6 (pyridoxine), B12 (cyanocobalmin), and folic acid. All the B vitamins except B12 are found in nuts, seeds, green vegetables, whole cereals, and wheat germs. B12 is the only vitamin not present in plant foods. Only tiny amounts of B12 are needed, and vegetarians usually get this from dairy products. If you are a vegan or a strict vegetarian who consumes few animal products, you need to incorporate a vitamin B12 supplement or B12-fortified foods into your diet. Nowadays, vitamin B12 is being added to soymilks, veggie burgers, and many breakfast cereals.

Vitamin C: All citrus fruits, most fresh fruits, vegetables, and leafy green vegetables.

Vitamin D: Humans can make this important vitamin in their skin when it is exposed to sunlight. This vitamin is not found in plant foods, but it is added to most dairy products.

Vitamin E: Most vegetable oils, whole-grain cereals, and eggs.

Vitamin K: Your body can absorb this vitamin from your intestines, as the bacteria in the gut synthesize it. All fresh vegetables and cereals can provide this vital vitamin too.

Vitamins: Their Food Sources and Functions

Name: Vitamin B1 (thiamin)

Functions: Improves metabolism, improves heart function, healthy nervous system

Dose: 1.5 mg

Source: Whole grains, legumes, organ meats, seeds, nuts, beef, fish, poultry, yeast, whole-grain breads, pasta, rice, soybeans

Deficiency: Thiamin deficiency is most commonly seen in alcoholics. A deficiency of thiamin can cause weakness, fatigue, psychosis, and central nervous system damage.

Toxicity: There is no known toxicity to thiamin.

Solubility: Water soluble

Antioxidant Activity: None

Name: Vitamin B2 (riboflavin)

Functions: Healthy skin, good vision, body growth, red blood cell production, improve metabolism

Dose: 1.7 mg

Source: Meat, eggs, legumes, nuts, green leafy vegetables, dairy products, poultry, fish

Deficiency: A deficiency in vitamin B2 can cause dry and cracked skin and sensitivity to bright light.

Toxicity: As with all other water-soluble vitamins, excess amounts are excreted by the body in the urine.

Solubility: Water soluble

Antioxidant Activity: None

Name: Vitamin B3 (niacin)

Functions: Metabolism, healthy skin, healthy nervous system, healthy digestive system

Dose: 20 mg

Source: Yeast, meats, eggs, liver, cereals, legumes, seeds, green leafy vegetables, fish, nuts, poultry, enriched grains, dairy products, veal, rice

Deficiency: A deficiency of niacin causes pellagra-inflamed skin, digestive problems, and mental impairment.

Toxicity: Large doses of niacin may cause liver damage and skin rashes.

Solubility: Water soluble

Antioxidant Activity: None

Name: Vitamin B5 (pantothenic acid)

Functions: Metabolism, energy production

Dose: 10 mg

Source: Whole grains, legumes, milk, eggs, liver

Deficiency: There are no known deficiencies of pantothenic acid.

Toxicity: Large doses can cause diarrhea.

Solubility: Water soluble

Antioxidant Activity: None

Name: Vitamin B6 (pyridoxine)

Functions: Metabolism, central nervous system function, formation of red blood cells, normal brain function, energy production

Dose: 2 mg

Source: Whole grains, legumes, meat, poultry, fish, nuts, green leafy vegetables, bananas, eggs, fortified breads, cereals

Deficiency: Anemia, dermatitis, conjunctivitis, somnolence, confusion, and neuropathy.

Toxicity: Large doses can cause nerve damage and numbness.

Solubility: Water soluble

Antioxidant Activity: None

Name: Vitamin B7 (biotin)

Functions: Metabolism, decrease stress, decrease anxiety, decrease insomnia, normal hair production and growth.

Dose: 300 mcg

Source: Liver, egg yolks, soy, cereals, yeast

Deficiency: Toxicity:

Solubility: Water soluble

Antioxidant Activity: None

Name: Vitamin B12 (cobalamin)

Functions: Development of red blood cells, maintenance of the central nervous system, metabolism

Dose: 6 mcg

Source: Meats, eggs, yeast, poultry, fish, dairy, beef liver, oysters

Deficiency: Deficiency of vitamin B12 is extremely rare. Pernicious anemia can develop from the inability to absorb vitamin B12.

Toxicity: None

Solubility: Water soluble

Antioxidant Activity: None

Name: Vitamin C (ascorbic acid)

Functions: An antioxidant, healthy gums, healthy teeth, increase iron absorption, production of collagen, promote wound healing, boost the immune system

Dose: 60 mg

Source: Fruits, berries, mangos, citrus fruits, tomatoes, peppers, broccoli, potatoes, green and yellow vegetables, melons, green peppers, green leafy vegetables, red peppers

Deficiency: A deficiency of vitamin C causes scurvy.

Toxicity: Excessive doses of vitamin C can lead to toxicity and possible kidney stones.

Solubility: Water soluble

Antioxidant Activity: None

Name: Vitamin D (choleacalciferol)

Functions: Regulates absorption of calcium and phosphorus, aids in development of healthy bones and teeth, healthy nervous system, healthy muscles

Dose: 400 IU

Source: Dairy, fish, liver, eggs, sunlight. Direct sunshine fifteen minutes a day is enough for vitamin D production.

Deficiency: A deficiency of vitamin D can cause soft, brittle bones and fractures.

Toxicity: Vitamin D is toxic in large doses, especially in children and pregnant women.

Solubility: Fat soluble

Antioxidant Activity: None

Name: Vitamin E (alpha and gamma tocopherol)

Functions: An antioxidant, protects red blood cells, protects cell membranes, protects lipoproteins

Dose: 30 IU

Source: Nuts, vegetables, seeds, wheat grains, wheat germ, green leafy vegetables, vegetable oil, corn, olives, corn oil, sunflower oil, soybean oil, cottonseed oil

Deficiency: There is no known dietary deficiency of vitamin E.

Toxicity: There are no known toxic effects of vitamin E.

Solubility: Fat soluble

Antioxidant Activity: None

Name: Folic Acid

Functions: Synthesis of DNA, normal growth, metabolism, reduces the risk of certain birth defects (especially spina bifida), red blood cell formation

Dose: 400 mcg

Source: Green leafy vegetables, liver, legumes, seeds, rice, pasta, dark green leafy vegetables, whole grains, citrus fruit, pumpkin, carrots, sweet potatoes, eggs, cheese

Deficiency: Folic acid deficiency may cause hemolytic and megaloblastic anemias, poor growth, graying hair, mouth ulcers, and peptic ulcers.

Toxicity: Toxicity from excessive folic acid intake does not normally occur.

Solubility: Water soluble

Antioxidant Activity: None

Name: Vitamin K

Functions: Normal blood clotting, growth, healthy bones

Dose: 80 mcg

Source: Liver, spinach, kale, broccoli, other dark green leafy vegetables, dairy, turnips, cabbages, cauliflower, avocados

Deficiency: Lack of vitamin K can slow clotting.

Toxicity: Large doses can cause anemia and a severe form of jaundice in infants.

Solubility: Fat soluble

Antioxidant Activity: None

List of Vitamins and Related Systems

Vitamin A (beta-carotene)

- Vision
- Growth
- Bones
- Healing
- Red blood cells

Vitamin B1 (thiamin)

- Nervous system function
- Mood
- Energy

Vitamin B2 (riboflavin)

- Energy
- Skin
- Vision

Vitamin B3 (niacin)

- Blood pressure
- Circulation
- Cholesterol
- Brain

Vitamin B5 (pantothenic acid)

- Energy
- Adrenal glands
- Menstruation

Vitamin B6 (pyridoxine)

- Brain
- Blood pressure
- Heart
- Mood
- Immune system

Vitamin B7 (biotin)

- Energy
- Sleep
- Hair

Vitamin B12 (cobalamin)

- Brain
- Red blood cells
- Energy
- Adrenal glands
- Cholesterol

Vitamin C (ascorbic acid)

- Immune system
- Healing
- Cholesterol

Vitamin D (choleacalciferol)

+ Bone formation

Vitamin E (alpha and gamma tocopherol)

+ Red blood cells

+ Immune system

+ Heart

+ Brain function

Vitamin K

+ Clotting

+ Bone growth

Folic Acid

+ Red blood cells

+ Energy

+ Sleep

Minerals

Minerals are elements that originate in the Earth's crust and hence vary with geographic locale. In addition, minerals may also be present in the water you drink (594). Plants absorb minerals from the soil. Minerals from plant sources may also vary from place to place, because soil mineral content varies geographically. Since minerals cannot be made by living organisms, most of the minerals in your diets come directly from plants or indirectly from animals that ingest these plants (594). Minerals perform a variety of functions in your body. Major minerals include calcium, iron, zinc, iodine, phosphorus, magnesium, copper, selenium, chromium, boron, and manganese.

List of Minerals

Boron

Food sources: fresh fruits, vegetables, nuts

Functions: strengthens the bones

Calcium

Food sources: green leafy vegetables, beans, nuts, seeds, soymilk

Functions: strengthens the bones, teeth, improves blood clotting

Chromium

Food sources: whole-grain breads, spices, and herbs

Functions: controls the blood-sugar levels, improves insulin response

Copper

Food sources: whole grains, dark green leafy vegetables, legumes

Functions: improves cardiovascular function (heart, arteries, and blood vessels), improves muscle function, strengthens the bones, improves nerve transmission, increases production of red blood cells, hair, and skin, improves metabolism

Iodine

Food sources: salt, yeast, vegetables, almonds, mushrooms

Functions: thyroid hormone, metabolism, growth, reproduction, nervous system, muscle, hair, skin

Iron

Food sources: dark green leafy vegetables, legumes, nuts and seeds, whole grains

Functions: increases red blood cells, improves immune system and energy level

Magnesium

Food sources: nuts, seeds, beans, avocados, bananas, dark green leafy vegetables, whole grains, soybeans

Functions: improves cell metabolism, improves muscle function, function of peripheral nervous system, strengthens the teeth, aids heart function

Manganese

Food sources: spinach, tea, whole-grain breads, raisins, blueberries, pineapples, legumes, nuts, dark green leafy vegetables

Functions: connective tissues, cholesterol, bones, blood-clotting factors, protein, metabolism

Phosphorous

Food sources: legumes, soybeans, nuts, seeds, bran

Functions: bones, teeth, growth, healing, central nervous system, peripheral nervous system, muscle, metabolism

Potassium

Food sources: fruits, vegetables, grains, potatoes, avocados, bananas, oranges, beans

Functions: central and peripheral nervous system, cell membrane, blood pressure, heartbeat

Selenium

Food sources: all vegetables grown in selenium-rich soil

Functions: antioxidant, protect against cancer, heart disease, pregnancy

Zinc

Food sources: nuts, seeds, beans, mushrooms, whole grains

Functions: prostate, metabolism, insulin, healing

Names and Sources of Antioxidants

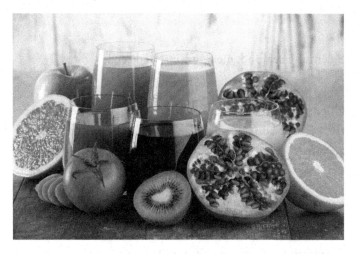

Following are major known antioxidants and their sources.

Vitamin A (beta-carotene): all colorful fruits and vegetables, carrots, kale, parsley, spinach, turnips, apricots, peaches

Vitamin C: oranges, grapefruits, tangerines, berries, broccoli, brussels sprouts, collards, guava, kale, turnip greens, sweet peppers, cabbage, cauliflower, spinach, watercress, melons

Vitamin E: unprocessed vegetable oils, whole grains, dark green leafy vegetables, nuts, legumes

Lycopene: tomatoes, watermelon, papaya, pink grapefruit, pink guava

Lutein: corn, egg yolks, fruits, broccoli, brussels sprouts, kale, cabbage, green beans, green peas, spinach, kiwifruit, honeydew melon

Zeaxanthin: egg yolks, vegetables, green beans, green peas

Selenium: seafood, meat, grains, and seeds

Coenzyme Q10: organ meats (especially hearts) are the richest sources; beef and chicken contain smaller amounts

Proanthocyanidins: grape seeds

Quercetin: onions, green tea, red wine

Turmeric: turmeric, curry

Ellagic acid: berries, pecans, walnuts, pomegranates

Hesperidin: oranges, tangelos, lemons

Glucose, Fructose, Sucrose: Are They the Same?

Glucose, fructose, and sucrose are unique, different molecules. Glucose and fructose are monosaccharides, while sucrose is a disaccharide composed of glucose and fructose linked via a weak bond. A molecule of sucrose can be broken down into a molecule of glucose and a molecule of fructose in the acidic environment of stomach or during digestion by the enzyme sucrose.

Cane sugar and beet sugar are both relatively pure sucrose, while honey is a mixture of different types of sugars, water, and small amounts of other compounds.

High-Fructose Corn Syrup

High-fructose corn syrup (HFCS) includes any of a group of corn syrups that has undergone enzymatic processing to convert its glucose into fructose and has then been mixed with pure corn syrup (100 percent glucose) to produce a desired sweetness. The most widely used varieties of high-fructose corn syrup are:

1. HFCS 55, which is commonly used in soft drinks, contains approximately 55 percent fructose and 45 percent glucose.

2. HFCS 42, which is commonly used in many processed foods and baked goods, contains 42 percent fructose and 58 percent glucose

Due to government subsidies of US corn and an import tariff on foreign sugar, high-fructose corn syrup has become very cost-efficient for many sweetener applications. HFCS is typically used as a sugar substitute in processed foods and beverages, including soft drinks, yogurt, industrially baked bread, cookies, and salad dressing.

It is believed that the highly processed substance is more harmful to humans than regular sugar, contributing to weight gain by affecting normal appetite functions (142–143). There are, however, scientific claims that HFCS is comparable to table sugar. Some studies by the American Medical Association suggest that it is unlikely that HFCS contributes more to obesity or other conditions than sucrose, but calls for further independent research on the subject (142–146).

Eliminate Bad Drinks Like Soda

It is important to realize that soda replaces healthier drinks. It is self-evident that if you drink soda, you cut the intake of important liquids like water, milk, and juices and deprive yourself from essential nutrients, vitamins, and minerals. It is better to drink water, tea, and pure fruit juice with pulp, which are rich in antioxidants and have been shown to protect the body from many health problems.

Soft drinks are extremely popular for several reasons. The most important one being that they can easily be purchased. They are also popular because they are heavily marketed. Billions and billions of dollars are spent on advertising sodas and marketing them everywhere, including fast-food chains, supermarket checkouts, café shops and restaurants, gas stations, and even schools.

Mistakenly, many people believe that soda drinks are best to quench their thirst. However, they are probably the worst drinks to quench your thirst. Soda drinks are a major source of caffeine in the American diet. By avoiding these soda drinks, you will eliminate unnecessary caffeine. There is much scientific evidence that high doses of caffeine can cause irritability, restlessness, insomnia, higher blood pressure, excessive urination and dehydration, irregular heartbeat, and other side effects (147–153). And because caffeine is a mildly addictive substance, kicking the soda habit can be difficult.

The fact that you are thirsty indicates that you are dehydrated; your body lacks fluids. To replenish the body with caffeinated drinks would cause more dehydration, since caffeine is a mild diuretic and causes more dehydration. So, when you drink a caffeinated soda to quench your thirst, you will actually become thirstier. Furthermore, as a direct result of dehydration, the body's production of saliva is severely reduced. Due to the lack of this important body fluid, which helps to neutralize acids, the acidic sodas can promote tooth decay.

Why You Should Stop Drinking Soda

There are many reasons you should give up soda. It is well documented that drinking carbonated, caffeinated, sugared, or artificially sweetened beverages are harmful to your body (154). Giving up or markedly reducing intake of soft drinks and switching to water can be one of the significant things you can do to improve your health.

Soda drinks chiefly consist of water and refined sugars, and there are no nutritionally beneficial components in soft drinks. Most people don't appreciate how many extra calories they consume in their drinks—especially soft drinks. The truth is that the empty calories in these drinks are partly responsible for the surge in obesity in America, most specifically in children. For example, a twelve-ounce can of Coca-Cola or Pepsi Cola contains thirty-nine grams of sugar, which is equal to one hundred forty calories. If you drink one a day for thirty days, that translates to more than a one pound weight gain!

Many scientific research studies have demonstrated experimentally that soft drinks are directly related to weight gain. Amazingly, the researchers have even calculated the direct relationship between soft drink consumption and body weight. This calculation points to an alarming 1.5 times risk of obesity for each additional soda drink consumed (154).

Based on another research study, reducing consumption of sugar-sweetened drinks can help reduce BMI in the heaviest teenagers (155).

As your BMI increases, the risk of developing diabetes does as well. In fact, drinking soda drinks not only increases your weight but also adversely affects your body's ability to process sugar. There is some agreement among scientists that the sugar/HFCS contents help explain why the number of Americans with type II diabetes has more than tripled from 6.5 million in 1980 to more than 21 million today. Researchers tracking more than fifty-one thousand women over eight years found that women who drank one or more sugary drinks a day gained more weight and were 80 percent more likely to develop type 2 diabetes than those who drank less than one a month (156, 157).

It is important to mention that consumption of fructose from its natural sources (fruits/fruit juices) is greatly different than HFCS. The HFCS is rapidly absorbed and, therefore, causes great fluctuations in blood sugar. As a result, it will put more strain on insulin-producing cells than other foods that are absorbed slower.

Physiologically, when sugar enters the bloodstream fast, the pancreas has to produce and release large amounts of insulin for the body to process it. It is believed by some researchers that the constant demands that a soda habit places on the pancreas may ultimately leave it unable to keep up with the body's need for insulin or become resistant to its action and may contribute to the risk of developing diabetes.

Interestingly, in a study conducted in young and middle-aged women, it was found that subjects who consumed a lot of fruit juice—which is high in natural fructose—were not at increased risk of diabetes, leading researchers to speculate that naturally occurring sugars may have different metabolic effects than added sugars. They also speculate that vitamins, minerals, fiber, and phytochemicals in fruit juices may have a protective effect against weight gain and diabetes, counterbalancing the adverse effects of sugar (158).

Risk of Osteoporosis

Osteoporosis is a major health issue in the United States. Some scientists believe that the culprit may be decreased intake of milk in the diet as a consequence of drinking sodas. Furthermore, other scientists believe that the acidity of colas may be weakening bones by promoting the loss of calcium (159–163).

Furthermore, a large amount of soda/cola consumption in children increases the risk factor for impaired calcification of their growing bones. These findings are disturbing, considering epidemiological studies clearly show that compared to the 1950s, when children drank three cups of milk for every one cup of sugary drinks, that ratio is reversed today: three cups of sugary drinks for every cup of milk (162).

Dental Decay and Erosion

The acidity of soda drinks can weaken and damage your teeth by dissolving the mineral content of the tooth enamel. There is some evidence that supports the notion that soft drinks are responsible for almost tripling the incidence of tooth decay (162). Soda's acidity makes it even worse for teeth than the solid sugar found in candy. Therefore, dentists recommend lesser intake of sodas between meals to prevent tooth decay.

The result of an interesting study at Purdue University supports the notion that people who drink sugary drinks/sodas don't feel as satiated as those who consume the same amount of calories in solid food. In this study, the researchers provided volunteers with four hundred fifty calories a day of either soda or jelly beans for a month and then switched them for the next month, while monitoring their total calories. Interestingly, during the phase of eating candy, the volunteers consumed less food and maintained their weight. During the soda phase, the volunteers ate more and gained.

Of course, even though the sugar in the soda drinks (liquid sugar) is a problem, the type of carbohydrate (sugar) used in the majority of soft drinks makes the damage and adverse effects even worse. There is some evidence that the sweeteners in sodas—HFCS—fail to suppress the production of a powerful hormone called ghrelin, which is produced and released by the stomach and stimulates appetite.

Simply put, when you consume good carbohydrates containing 100 percent glucose, such as the starch found in rice, potatoes, bread, and pasta, they trigger the hormones that help you regulate appetite and fat storage. On the other hand, carbohydrates derived from HFCS, these important hormones are not released adequately. As a result, your body never gets the message that you are satiated and should stop eating. It is self-evident that after drinking a large glass of soda, which may contain several hundred of calories, your body feels no fuller than if you'd just drank the same amount of water.

There may be some evidence in the medical literature to support the notion that cola beverages can increase the risk of kidney problems, more so than non-cola sodas. For example, two different research studies demonstrated that large quantities of cola result in enhanced kidney stone formation. It is believed that because of their acidity and radical mineral imbalances, your body must buffer the acidity of soft drinks by taking calcium from your bones. This increases the amount of calcium in your urine. In combination with some degree of dehydration from caffeinated drinks, calcium in the urine is increased to the point of saturation and precipitation, which, over time, leads to forming kidney stones (163, 164).

Disturbingly, in another study, a team of researchers compared the dietary habits of individuals with chronic kidney disease and healthy people. The team found that drinking two or more colas a day was linked to a twofold risk of chronic kidney disease (165).

Higher Blood Pressure and Metabolic Syndrome Risk Factor

In a short-term study, overconsumption of fructose, particularly in the form of soft drinks, acutely elevates blood pressure in healthy young humans. Whether high fructose consumption is stressful to your body is a question that needs further study (166).

Liver Disease

The effect of a long-term nutritional intake and the risk of developing nonalcoholic fatty liver disease were studied in a population-based study by a group of researchers. According to their study, there is evidence that consumption of too many soft drinks puts you under increased risk for liver disease known as cirrhosis, which is similar to what chronic alcoholics often develop (167).

Another important issue regarding cola drinks is the amount of phosphoric acid they contain. The phosphoric acid from soda drinks competes with the hydrochloric acid of the stomach and affects its digestive functions, which are important for proper digestion. When the digestive juices become ineffective, food remains in the stomach longer, causing indigestion, gassiness, or bloating.

Last but not least, there are some health concerns related to a common preservative added to the soft drinks. Sodium benzoate, or E211, is used in large quantities to prevent mold in soft drinks (168). One of the concerns is possible cell damage, most specifically related to the ability of this preservative to switch off vital parts of DNA. A research group from Sheffield University, which has been studying sodium benzoate for almost a decade, has found that this preservative seriously damages living cells. According to the lead researcher, these chemicals have the ability to cause severe damage to mitochondrial to the point that they totally inactivate it: they knock it out altogether. Of course, it is self-evident that you cannot avoid all the above mentioned problems by just drinking calorie- and caffeine-free cola.

At this point, even though we have much better understandings of the macronutrients and micronutrients, we still need to learn about the vital and necessary tools to achieve desired health and nutrition and ultimately weight management.

In this section, we review some of the important and necessary tools for proper nutrition and weight management. These include:

Metabolism
Basal metabolic rate (BMR)
Body mass index (BMI)

You'll also learn how to calculate your BMR and BMI.

Metabolism

Metabolism is the sum of all the processes that take place within your body that enable its continued growth and functioning. Metabolism converts ingested food and energy stored as fat into energy or calories required for the basal metabolic rate (BMR) (see pages 00–00). If your intake of calories exceed your BMR, the excess calories are stored as fat for future use. In simple terms, if you have a faster metabolism, you burn calories more efficiently and store less fat. If you have a slower metabolism, you burn calories less efficiently and, therefore, store more calories as fat. Metabolism includes two groups of chemical reactions in the body. Anabolism is building up processes, in contrast to catabolism, which is the breaking down processes in the cells of your body.

There are three components to your metabolic rate:

1   Base metabolic rate, or BMR.

2   Physical activity.

3   Thermal effect of food, or TEF.

TEF refers to the fact that when you are convert energy from one form to another; it is never 100 percent efficient. So, by eating, you are spending energy to convert it to calories.

Your metabolic rate is the rate and efficiency with which your body performs and achieves these metabolic tasks.

Mordechai S. Nosrati, MD

Basal Metabolic Rate (BMR)

BMR is a scientific name for the minimum number of calories needed to maintain bodily functions at rest, but not asleep, and at room temperature. These bodily functions are needed for survival. They include respiration, heartbeat, perspiration, and maintenance of normal body temperature and brain activities.

Your BMR typically accounts for approximately 60 percent to 70 percent of your daily caloric requirements. Age and sex can affect the BMR: your BMR will usually peak at the age of twenty and gradually decline. The BMR difference between a twenty-year-old person and a sixty-year-old person can be up to 10 percent, or approximately 2 percent per decade of aging above age twenty. These differences are mostly due to inactivity and loss of muscle tissue.

Calculating Your BMR

There are two ways you can calculate your BMR. One method is the Harris Benedict formula, explained on page 00. An alternative and easier way to calculate your BMR and calorie needs is to multiply your body weight in pounds by ten. This will roughly give you your BMR. For example, if you weigh 150 pounds, your BMR is 150 x 10 = 1,500 calories.

Multiply the BMR by the activity multiplier. Activity multiplier is a factor by which BMR increases. The more active you are the higher your activity multiplier. The following is the activity provider for each level of activity.

Activity Multiplier
Sedentary = BMR × 1.2 (little or no exercise, desk job)
Lightly active = BMR × 1.375 (light exercise/sports 1–3 days/wk)
Moderately active = BMR × 1.55 (moderate exercise/sports 3–5 days/wk)
Very active = BMR × 1.725 (hard exercise/sports 6–7 days/wk)
Extremely active = BMR × 1.9 (hard daily exercise/physical job)

This simple calculation yields values close to the more sophisticated calculation used in the Harris Benedict formula.

Example:

If a 150-pound man does very little activity, his daily calorie needs in order to maintain his 150 pounds would be:

1,500 calories BMR x 1.2 factor

Thus, he needs 1,800 calories to maintain his weight.

If the same 150-pound man does light exercise, his daily calorie needs would be:

1,500 calories BMR x 1.4 factor

Thus, he needs 2,100 calories to maintain his weight.

Body Mass Index (BMI)

BMI is the most widely used diagnostic tool to identify weight problems within a population. It is also one of the most accurate ways to find out if extra weight can put you at greater health risks. BMI takes into account your weight and height to determine your total body fat. Someone with a BMI of 26 is about 20 percent overweight. This usually carries a moderate health risk. A BMI of 30 or higher is considered obese. A BMI of less than 18.5 is usually considered as underweight (169). The most immediate problem with underweight is that it might be secondary to, or symptomatic of, an underlying disease. Unexplained weight loss requires professional medical diagnosis.

Simply put, the higher your BMI, the higher the risk of developing additional health problems. These include heart disease, diabetes, and high blood pressure, which are all linked to being overweight. Use the BMI chart to find your current BMI and your optimal weight for a healthier BMI.

BMI Based on Weight (lbs.) and Height (ft.) (170)

Weight (lbs) → Height ↓	100	105	110	115	120	125	130	135	140	145	150	155	160	165	170	175	180	185	190	195	200	205	210	215	220	225	230	235	240	245	250
5'0"	20	21	21	22	23	24	25	26	27	28	29	30	31	32	33	34	35	36	37	38	39	40	41	42	43	44	45	46	47	48	49
5'1"	19	20	21	22	23	24	25	26	26	27	28	29	30	31	32	33	34	35	36	37	38	39	40	41	42	43	43	44	45	46	47
5'2"	18	19	20	21	22	23	24	25	26	27	27	28	29	30	31	32	33	34	35	36	37	37	38	39	40	41	42	43	44	45	46
5'3"	18	19	19	20	21	22	23	24	25	26	27	27	28	29	30	31	32	33	34	35	35	36	37	38	39	40	41	42	43	43	44
5'4"	17	18	19	20	21	21	22	23	24	25	26	27	27	28	29	30	31	32	33	33	34	35	36	37	38	39	39	40	41	42	43
5'5"	17	17	18	19	20	21	22	22	23	24	25	26	27	27	28	29	30	31	32	32	33	34	35	36	37	37	38	39	40	41	42
5'6"	16	17	18	19	19	20	21	22	23	23	24	25	26	27	27	28	29	30	31	31	32	33	34	35	36	36	37	38	39	40	40
5'7"	16	16	17	17	18	20	20	21	22	22	23	24	25	26	26	27	28	29	30	30	31	32	33	34	34	35	36	37	38	38	39
5'8"	15	16	17	17	18	19	20	21	21	22	23	24	24	25	26	27	27	28	29	30	30	31	32	33	33	34	35	36	36	37	38
5'9"	15	16	16	17	18	18	19	20	21	21	22	23	24	24	25	26	27	27	28	29	30	30	31	32	32	33	34	35	35	36	37
5'10"	14	15	16	16	17	18	19	19	20	21	22	22	23	24	24	25	26	27	27	28	29	29	30	31	32	32	33	34	34	35	36
5'11"	14	15	15	16	17	17	18	19	20	20	21	22	22	23	24	24	25	26	26	27	28	29	29	30	31	31	32	33	33	34	35
6'0"	14	14	15	16	16	17	18	18	19	20	20	21	22	22	23	24	24	25	26	26	27	28	28	29	30	31	31	32	33	33	34
6'1"	13	14	15	15	16	16	17	18	18	19	20	20	21	22	22	23	24	24	25	26	26	27	28	28	29	30	30	31	32	32	33
6'2"	13	13	14	15	15	16	17	17	18	19	19	20	21	21	22	22	23	24	24	25	26	26	27	28	28	29	30	30	31	31	32
6'3"	12	13	14	14	15	16	16	17	17	18	19	19	20	21	21	22	22	23	24	24	25	26	26	27	27	28	29	29	30	31	31
6'4"	12	13	13	14	15	15	16	16	17	18	18	19	19	20	21	21	22	23	23	24	24	25	26	26	27	27	28	29	29	30	30

Food Groups & Food Pyramids

Food groups refers to a method of classification for the various foods that we consume in our everyday lives, based on the nutritional properties of these types of foods and their location in a hierarchy of nutrition. As we have discussed, consuming certain types and proportions of foods from the different categories has a positive health benefits. Therefore, these foods are recommended by most guides to healthy eating as one of the most important ways to achieve a healthy lifestyle through diet. There are six major food components:

1. Carbohydrates
2. Proteins
3. Fats/oils
4. Fibers
5. Minerals
6. Vitamins

However, there are ten basic food groups which provide the six basic components essential and required for optimal human health, nutrition, and growth. The ten basic components of the Diet of L.O.V.E. Program are as follows:

1. Fruits
2. Vegetables, herbs, spices, and prebiotics
3. Dried nuts and seeds, spices
4. Meat, poultry, and fish
5. Grains
6. Dried beans and lentils
7. Dairy products and probiotics
8. Oils/fats
9. Water, purified, not bottled preferred
10. Natural sweeteners

Food Groups and some Examples

1. Fruits [Apples, apricots, bananas, dates, grapes, oranges, grapefruit, grapefruit juice, mangoes, melons, peaches, pineapples, raisins, strawberries, tangerines, and 100 percent fruit juice with pulp]

2. Vegetables, herbs, spices, and prebiotics [Broccoli, carrots, collards, green beans, green peas, kale, spinach, squash, sweet potatoes, tomatoes, tarragon basil, mint, rosemary, etc.]

3. Dried nuts and seeds, spices [kidney beans, lentils, split peas, chickpeas, pinto beans, black beans, etc.]

4. Meat, poultry, and fish [Lean meats, beef, pork, game meats, chicken, turkey, fish, shellfish]

5. Grains [whole-wheat bread and rolls, whole-wheat pasta, English muffin, pita bread, bagel, cereals, grits, oatmeal, brown rice, etc.]

6. Dried beans and lentils [Almonds, hazelnuts, mixed nuts, peanuts, walnuts, sunflower seeds]

7. Dairy products and probiotics [Fat-free or low-fat milk and milk products, low-fat or reduced fat cheese, fat-free or low-fat regular or frozen yogurt and kefir and cultured yogurt]

8. Oils/fats [olive oil, grape seed oil, walnut oil, sunflower oil, corn oil, almond oil, etc.]

9. Water [mineral water, purified not bottled preferred]

10. Natural sweeteners [honey, Stevia]

Approximate calorie content of one serving for each different food group

1. Vegetables: contain 25 calories and 5 grams of carbohydrate.

2. Low-fat dairy products: contain 100 calories per serving.

3. Fruits: contain 15 grams of carbohydrate and 60 calories.

4. Very lean proteins (1 gram of fat per serving) have 35 calories per serving.

5. Lean proteins (2-3 grams of fat per serving) have 55 calories per serving.

6. Medium-fat proteins (5 grams of fat per serving) have 75 calories per serving.

7. Fats (5 grams) contain 45 calories

My Optimum Plate vs. My Plate

Interestingly, there are various systems of dividing foods into groups to develop models of optimum nutrition for humans. Among these systems are the US Department of Agriculture's (USDA) program titled My Pyramid, the Canadian Government's Canada's Food Guide, and the United Kingdom Food Standards Agency. Most recently the iconic Food Pyramid/My Pyramid has been replaced by the USDA's new food icon called My Plate. The new symbol looks like a dinner plate that is divided into four wedges. Half of the sections on the plate will be for fruits and vegetables. Two of those wedges are filled with fruits and vegetables, one contains protein, and the fourth has whole grains. Beside the plate is a smaller circle—representing low-fat dairy allowance. This new logo, at a cost of about $2 million to develop and promote, is meant to educate Americans about new federal dietary guidelines. However, there are some problems associated with this simple presentation of dietary intake.

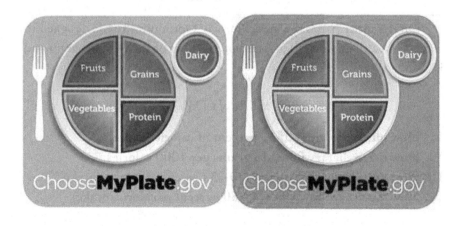

Problems with the MyPlate Icon

MyPlate is supposedly designed to educate Americans on how to adopt healthier diet at a time when more than 30 percent of children and more than 70 percent of adults in the United States are overweight or obese. According to the USDA, the new tool emphasizes which types of food groups to add more of to your diet, such as fruits, vegetables, protein, and whole grains, while reducing others like sodium and sugary drinks. However, the followings are the major problems with the MyPlate.

1. Just like the old food pyramid, MyPlate does not differentiate between healthier and unhealthier fats. In fact, fats aren't even mentioned.

2. Reduction in sodium and refined sugar is never clearly expressed via the plate!

3. Even though MyPlate is very simple, however, it is very vague. This simplicity is not an improvement, rather it is incomplete and confusing and misleading. Calories are not mentioned on the plate or the website accompanying it. For example what is the size of the plate? What kinds of grains and proteins should be consumed? What is the percentage of calories from each food group?

4. No guidelines warning Americans about avoiding artificial sweeteners, artificial colors, high-fructose corn syrup, and preservatives like nitrates and nitrites.

On the other hand, the model for My Optimum Plate is designed to promote health and nutrition based on the Diet of L.O.V.E. program and is as follows:

Composition of Diet of L.O.V.E. Program

I.   How much protein? (10-35 percent of calorie intake)
II. How much dietary fiber? 15 grams per 1000 calories
III. How much total dietary fat? (20-35 percent of calorie intake)
IV. How much carbohydrate? (45-60 percent of calorie intake)

I. How much protein? (10–35 percent)

In general, it's recommended that 10–35 percent of your daily calories come from protein. (Approximately 25 percent)

1 cup of milk has 8 grams of protein

A 3-ounce piece of meat has about 21 grams of protein

1 cup of dry beans has about 16 grams of protein

An 8-ounce container of yogurt has about 11 grams of protein

II. How much dietary fiber?

It's recommended that you get 15 grams of dietary fiber for every 1,000 calories that you consume each day. If you need 2,000 calories each day, you should try to include 30 grams of dietary fiber.

III. How much *total* dietary fat?

The *Dietary Guidelines for Americans 2005* recommend that Americans keep their total fat intake within certain limits. This limit is defined as a percentage of your total calorie needs. The range is minimum 20 percent to maximum 35 percent of calories from total fat.

Trans Fat (**reduce greatly**)

Saturated Fat (**reduce greatly**)

Cholesterol (**reduce greatly**)

Polyunsaturated Fats and Monounsaturated Fats (**major portion of the recommended daily fat intake**)

IV. How much carbohydrate?

It is recommended that 45 to 65 percent of the calories as carbohydrates. Of course this is mainly complex unrefined unprocessed carbohydrates

V. How much water?

You need at least eight glasses of water intake to maintain a good hydration. It should be emphasized that in certain circumstances the amount of water intake should be adjusted accordingly. For example when you are in hot climates, or when running a fever, or increasing your physical activity, you need to take in more water. Simply drink fluid while doing the activity and drink several glasses of water or other fluid after the physical activity is completed. Furthermore, when you are participating in vigorous physical activity, it's important to drink before you even feel thirsty.

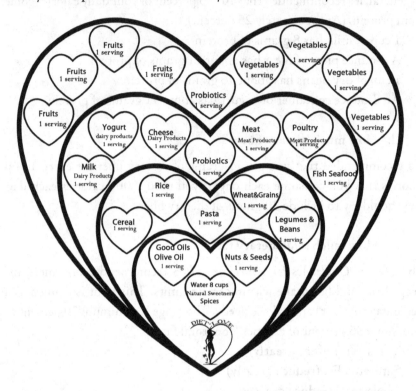

First Level

4 servings of Fruits (first level)
4 servings of Vegetables (first level)
1 serving of Prebiotic (first level)

Second Level

3 servings of Dairy (second level)
1 serving of Probiotic (second level)
3 serving of Meat, Poultry, and Fish (second level)

Third Level

4 servings of Grains (third level)
1 serving of Dried Legumes (third level)

Fourth Level

1 serving of Oils/Fats (fourth level)
1 serving of Nuts/Seeds about a handful (third level)
8 servings of water and/or healthy drinks (third level)

Examples:

Grains (4 servings a day)

One serving of grains includes
1 slice whole-wheat bread,
1 ounce (oz.) dry cereal, or
1/2 cup cooked cereal, rice, or pasta

Vegetables (4 servings a day)

One serving includes
1 cup raw leafy green vegetables
1/2 cup cut-up raw or cooked vegetables

Fruits (4 servings a day)

One serving includes
1 medium fruit or
1/2 cup fresh, frozen, or canned fruit
1 cup of 100 percent fruit juice with pulp or 1/2 cup of fruit juice (one serving of fruit is allowed per day)

Dairy (3 servings a day)

One serving includes
1 cup 1% or 2% milk
1 cup yogurt
1 1/2 oz. cheese

Lean Meat, Poultry, and Fish (3 servings a day)

One serving includes

> 2 oz. cooked skinless poultry, seafood or lean meat,
> 2 eggs, or
> 2 oz. canned tuna or fish

Nuts, Seeds (1 serving a day)

One serving includes
1/3 cup (1 1/2 oz.) nuts
2 tablespoons seeds

Dried Beans and Legumes (1 serving a day)

One serving includes;
1/2 cup cooked beans
1/2 cup cooked peas or lentils

Fats/Oils (2 to 3 servings a day)

One serving includes
3 teaspoons of olive oil
3 tablespoons low-fat mayonnaise (made with better quality oil)
12 tablespoons of salad dressing (made with 1 part olive or walnut oil in 3 parts balsamic vinegar or lemon/lime juice).
Note: Avoid saturated fat and trans fat

Sweets (1 serving per day)

One serving includes
2 tablespoons honey,
2 tablespoons jelly or jam,
1/2 cup of frozen low-sugar yogurt or sorbet
Note: Artificial sweeteners Splenda and Stevia may be used additionally in moderate amounts to help satisfy your sweet cravings

Water/Liquids (minimum 8 servings per day)

One serving includes
An 8-oz. glass of sparkling water
An 8-oz. glass of tap water (filtered)

An 8-oz. glass of lemonade drink (with Splenda or Stevia)
An 8-oz. glass of iced tea/herbal tea/green tea
Note: With increased activity and in certain situations (fever, hot climate, and diarrhea) water intake should be adjusted upward accordingly.

Prebiotics (at least 1 serving per day)

Dietary sources of prebiotics include soybeans, Jerusalem artichoke, jicama, and chicory root, raw oats, unrefined wheat, unrefined barley and yacón. Additionally, dandelion greens, raw garlic, raw leek, raw onion, cooked onion, raw asparagus, raw wheat bran, whole-wheat flour can be used in their respective food group to ensure probiotic intake.

Probiotics (at least 1 serving per day)

Probiotic dairy products can be used to ensure delivery of healthy probiotic microbes into your gut.

Chapter Three

L of L.O.V.E.

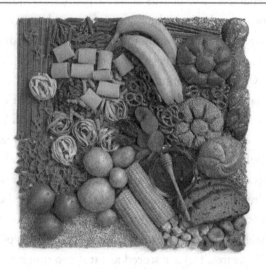

L Stands for Low-Calorie Diet: It Is the Number of Calories

Caloric Balance, Weight Loss, and Weight Control

Caloric balance is the most important and essential part of any successful diet. It is impossible to lose weight if you are not in negative caloric balance.

Caloric balance is the difference between calorie intake from food or drinks (calories in) and calories burned by metabolism and daily activities (calories out).

Caloric Balance = Calories In – Calories Out

In other words, any weight loss is the consequence of a negative caloric balance—the difference between calorie intake (energy intake) and calorie loss (energy expenditure).

Do Carbohydrates Make You Fat?

No. There is a myth propagated by the proponents of certain fad diets that starchy foods make you fat. They wrongly teach dieters that they should avoid foods like pasta, bread, and other carbohydrate-rich foods if they want to lose weight. There is not even a shred of truth to this claim. The whole claim that eating a lot of carbohydrates makes you produce too much insulin, and ultimately makes you insulin resistant, is not true. They further claim that because of this state of insulin resistance, your body has to pump more insulin, and the high insulin levels convert calories into fat. It is too naive to state that only foods rich in carbohydrate stimulates insulin production. The truth is that calories lead to weight gain, not the carbohydrates. Calories do count!

So, don't blame carbohydrates and the starchy foods alone. It is a fact that eating more calories than you burn and require will lead to weight gain no matter what the food type. It is absolutely not correct that eating a balanced carbohydrate diet makes you store fat easier. Calories in minus calories out dictates weight loss or gain. Since all types of food stimulate the release of insulin, it is not accurate to say that your body stores fat only when foods high in carbohydrates are eaten. The fundamental rule of human physiology and biochemistry dictates that all types of nutrients (protein, carbohydrates, fat) are stored as fat if too much is eaten. Simply put, if you take in more calories than you burn in a day, all those unburned calories will be stored as fat. Overall, it does not matter what percentage of those calories came from fat, protein, or carbohydrates.

However, a word of caution is needed to emphasize that balanced nutrition necessitates avoiding extremes in any specific food groups or nutrients. It is a scientific fact that obesity is what makes the cells in your body less sensitive to insulin, not your food choices (171–174). In fact, insulin resistance runs in families, and weight loss combined with increased physical activity can reduce its negative and dangerous effects. Insulin resistance increases the risk of heart disease, diabetes, and high blood pressure as part of a metabolic syndrome. Therefore, any kind of weight reduction and exercise can help increase a body's cell sensitivity to insulin.

Another important point to remember is that when you are anxious or depressed, your body craves more carbohydrates. That's because carbohydrates raise your body's levels of phenylethylamine and serotonin, the feel-good brain chemicals. (This may be one reason many of our "comfort foods" are high in carbohydrates.) When levels of these brain chemicals return to normal, the cycle is repeated, leading to an overeating syndrome.

Whole grains, beans, fruits, and vegetables should constitute a major portion of your daily caloric intake. They contain many of the macronutrients and micronutrients necessary for a healthy body. These nutrients include fiber, vitamins, and minerals. Eating high-fiber foods in combination with more good carbohydrates and starches can fill you up and reduce your fat intake.

Calories Do Count

If you seriously desire to lose weight and get into shape, you should remember this simple rule: you have to burn more calories than you consume. This is based on the laws of physics and life. Calories do count, no matter what other diet programs tell you.

Remember this fact: In order to maintain your weight you have to increase your level of physical activity (the amount of calories burned) more than the amount of calorie you eat. Otherwise, you will accumulate the extra calories as fat!

Imagine you want to lose ten pounds of fat. Since each pound of fat contains thirty-five hundred calories, this would equal thirty-five thousand calories. Now, if you reduce your caloric intake to five hundred calories less than the number of calories you burn every day, you could lose the ten pounds of fat in approximately seventy days! This can be done several different ways. You can reduce the number of calories you consume and not increase your activity level, you can maintain the number of calories consumed and increase your activity level, or you can reduce daily calorie intake and increase your activity level.

$$35,000 \div 500 = 70 \text{ days needed to lose } 35,000$$
calories at 500 calories per day!

Caloric Restriction Is Essential, Not Carbohydrate Restriction

Caloric restriction is an essential component of any successful weight-loss program. It is important to note that I am not talking about carbohydrate restriction. But how much caloric restriction is enough? Some people restrict calorie consumption too much too soon. There is a myth that sudden caloric restriction will shock the body into burning fat quicker. The body adapts to the caloric restriction by decreasing the metabolism, and it does not force increased fat burning at all! This is a natural defense against starvation and death and improves chance of survival in the time of famine or lack of food. Simply put, restricting calories too much will only result in a lowered metabolism as the body burns protein from lean muscle.

It is a well-known fact that people who restrict calories too much seek more food to satisfy their stronger appetite. I am sure you have the common experience of struggling with food cravings when starting a diet or fast. With these factors in mind, it is essential that caloric restriction is a gradual process developed over many months, not something done in a week or two. True caloric restriction is also more effective when nutritionally dense foods such as nuts and seeds are eaten in small and frequent meals—such as intake of only a handful of almonds or other nuts every day. A diet void of nutrient-dense foods may only cause further cravings and a greater appetite.

Therefore, restricting calories by eating healthy, low-calorie meals in smaller portions and more frequently (grazing) is the best way to lose weight permanently.

How Much Calorie Restriction Is Too Much?

The total number of calories should be restricted slowly and gradually. Total daily calories should not be fewer than an average of eleven hundred to twelve hundred calories per day for women and fourteen hundred to fifteen hundred for men. If you restrict your calories to fewer than one thousand, it may lead to health problems and nutritional deficiencies. It also causes fatigue and a lack of vitality.

Dangers of Very-Low-Calorie Diets

These fad diets are nothing more than starvation diets. The total caloric intake is about five hundred to six hundred calories for women and six hundred to eight hundred calories for men. These diets are dangerous and extremely hard to follow. There is a constant sense of hunger, which can increase your stress level, not to mention dangerous deficiencies in a number of macronutrients and micronutrients. This almost constant hunger can lead to hypoglycemia and, ultimately, bingeing. Even though you may see a very dramatic weight loss in the beginning, very low-calorie diets do not result in long-term loss. These dangerous diets often send dieters into a cycle of quick weight loss followed by a "rebound" weight gain once normal eating resumes. It is estimated that less than 5 percent of dieters actually keep weight off in the long run (175). It is not healthy to lose more than a pound per week. You should only attempt to follow a very-low-calorie diet if you are severely obese and then only under direct supervision of a physician.

Calculate Your Basal Metabolic Rate (Alternate Way) to Calculate Your Daily Caloric Needs

There is another method of calculating your BMR which some people may prefer. This alternate way basically gives you the same result as the previously mention method mentioned in chapter 2. As it was explained there, the minimum number of calories needed to maintain bodily function at rest is the basal metabolic rate (BMR). It measures the calorie expenditure at rest, not sleep, and at room temperature. To find out your daily caloric need, you first have to calculate your BMR. You can easily calculate your BMR.

1. Divide body weight in pounds by 2.2 to convert pounds to kilograms.

2. Multiply by factor 1.0 if you are a male, and 0.9 if you are a female.

3. Multiply the result by 24 (hours in a day) to calculate the daily calories.

This gives your BMR, or basic expenditure of calories, in a twenty-four-hour period. This is the *minimum* number of calories you need per day.

Example:

BMR calculation for a 220-pound male is as follows:
$220 \div 2.2 \times 1.0 \times 24 = 2{,}400$ calories per day

BMR calculation for a 110-pound female is as follows:

110 ÷ 2.2 x 0.9 x 24 = 1,080 calories per day

High-Protein Diets Can Hurt Your Kidneys

When your liver metabolizes proteins, they are broken down into their smallest constituents—amino acids—and waste products called blood urea nitrogen. Eating too much protein is believed to put too much strain on the body's ability to deal with waste products, particularly in people who already have a kidney problem. Each of your kidneys is made up of approximately one million tiny filters, which function in concert to clean waste products from your blood. A high-protein diet causes an increase in the pressure within these tiny filters. The high pressure in the filters causes them to scar and fail. When kidneys fail, you will need dialysis, and possibly a transplant, to survive.

Many nutritionists, health-care professionals, and medical societies, including the American Kidney Fund (AKF), have echoed this warning and are concerned about the popularity of high-protein, low-carbohydrate diets (176–178). Diets that emphasize a high intake of protein, place a significant strain on the kidneys. High-protein, low-carbohydrate diets are promoted on the myth that your body handles and metabolizes carbohydrates first and proteins last. Therefore, this supposed carbohydrate starvation forces your body to utilize and burn fat instead. Furthermore, it is presumed that high protein intake decreases hunger, so you eat less food.

Other concerns are that diets too high in protein are accompanied by a serious deficiency in the consumption of fiber, essential vitamins, and antioxidants from fruit and vegetables. They are also associated with a loss of calcium, which can weaken your bones. When you eat a high-protein diet, you jeopardize your health. High protein consumption, especially of animal protein, can result in many chronic diseases, including heart disease, stroke, osteoporosis, kidney disease, and kidney stones. The consumption of too much animal and saturated fat, which often occurs in a high-protein diet, can increase the risk of heart disease. It is a fact that our body needs protein, but too much of a good thing is not always good.

The average American diet contains approximately twice as much protein as is actually required by your body to function properly. So, if high-protein diets such as Atkins and similar programs are right, all Americans should be losing weight. And that isn't the case.

It is estimated that some people on high-protein diets consume up to four times the amount of protein their body needs. People with mild to severe kidney dysfunction should be careful to moderate their overall intake of meat. In addition, everyone should very carefully consider the risks and benefits before starting an Atkins-type diet.

Not All Proteins Are the Same: Eat Plant-Based Proteins

Plant-based proteins, like those found in soy, lower LDL (the bad) cholesterol and raise HDL (the good) cholesterol. This prevents the build up of arterial plaque, which leads to atherosclerosis (hardening of the arteries) and heart disease, thus reducing the risk of heart attack and stroke. The amount and type of protein in your diet also has an important impact on calcium absorption and excretion. Vegetable-protein diets enhance calcium retention in the body and result in less excretion of calcium in the urine. This reduces the risk of osteoporosis and kidney problems; kidney disease is far less common in people who eat a vegetable-based diet than it is in people who eat an animal-based diet (179). By replacing animal protein with vegetable protein and replacing saturated fat with unsaturated fat—like that found in olive and canola oils—you can avoid the pitfalls of the typical high-protein diet. You will be able to improve your health and regulate your weight while enjoying a vast array of delicious, nutritionally dense, high-fiber foods.

So, How Much Protein Does Your Body Really Need?

According to the American Heart Association and the National Institutes of Health, as little as fifty to sixty grams (two to three ounces) of protein is enough for most adults. This breaks down to about 10 percent to 12 percent of total calories (each ounce is equal to twenty-eight grams).

Here are examples of amounts of protein in food:

+ One cup of milk has eight to nine grams of protein.
+ Every ounce of lean meat, poultry, or fish provides seven grams of protein.

+ One cup of dry beans/legumes has about sixteen grams of protein.

+ Eight ounces of yogurt has about ten grams of protein.

+ A half cup of cooked beans provides seven grams of protein.

+ One ounce of cheese, one egg, or two egg whites provide seven grams of protein.

+ One cup of low-fat milk or yogurt provides seven grams of protein.

+ One serving of grain products (e.g., a slice of whole-wheat bread) provides three grams of protein.

Your body only needs 0.36 grams of protein per pound of body weight. To calculate the exact amount you need, multiply your ideal weight by 0.36. This will give you your optimum daily protein requirement in grams.

How Many Calories Are Enough?

The number of calories you need depends on several factors. The most important of these are your height, weight, age, gender, and physical activity level. The requirement can be changed with certain diseases or health issues. For example, in cases of severe illness—whether acute or chronic—or during pregnancy, the requirement needs to be adjusted upward.

On average, women require fewer calories than men. One can calculate calorie needs accurately by taking into consideration the two major calorie components: BMR and level of physical activity.

It is very important for you to know how many calories your body needs to function at rest. This is your BMR, and instructions on how to derive it have already been provided. Then you need to increase the second component by increasing your level of physical activity. This will guarantee that you will achieve a negative calorie balance.

Total Caloric Restriction

Caloric restriction is the only reliable way to increase your life span (180–183). With caloric restriction, your body produces lower levels of free radicals in your cells' power plant—the mitochondria. Caloric restriction also reduces serum glucose and insulin levels, thereby decreasing the formation of harmful products. These harmful products are by-products created when glucose cross-links with body proteins, such as collagen in the blood vessels. When these harmful products accumulate in the body, they can have a number of dangerous effects, including the creation of more inflammatory products and suppression of the immune response. When animals are calorie restricted, they show evidence of decreased production of free radicals and improved antioxidant defenses.

Metabolic Needs and Calorie Usage

Your BMR is the number of calories your body requires to maintain life and keep your organs and tissues in working order. On average, this accounts for 60 percent of all calories consumed. All other calories are used to meet our additional energy needs based on our level of physical activity. Your age, genes, percentage of muscle in your body, muscle-to-fat ratio, and activity level determine your metabolic rate.

Some people have a faster metabolism: it is in your genes. But it is not the only determinant. As you age, your decreases. As I have mentioned, it decreases by approximately 2 percent each decade. The more muscle you have, the higher your metabolism. Muscles are approximately eight times more metabolically active and demanding than fats. So, the greater your muscle mass, the faster your metabolic rate. Your level of activity is a major determinant of your metabolic rate.

How to Raise Metabolism

The good news is that even if your metabolic rate is genetically slow, it can be raised. There are several ways that this can be accomplished. The safest and most effective way to raise your metabolism is to increase your physical activity or exercise. The harder you work, the faster your metabolic rate. You should regularly perform aerobic exercises. Aerobic exercises are activities that make your heart beat faster and make you breathe heavier. Muscle-building exercises are also useful. The more muscle your body has, the more metabolically active it is.

A balanced diet is necessary. Make sure you eat regularly (three meals a day) and most specifically, eat breakfast. Eating typically wastes a modest amount of energy as heat due to the energy required for mastication (chewing) and digestion. This is called the thermic effect of food, or TEF. You can increase your TEF by eating small, frequent meals containing mostly proteins and carbohydrates. Unfortunately, eating fat generates virtually no TEF. Your body stores excess dietary fat directly as body fat, so there is no need to convert it.

A word of caution: eating more food is not a way to burn calories. To benefit from the TEF and ensure that your body burns calories willingly, eat breakfast and then eat regularly throughout the day. You should eat when you are hungry. Do not wait till you are overly hungry, as this can cause you to overeat easily. Never stuff yourself.

Exercise burns calories. Even after you stop exercising, the effect continues. So, your body will burn calories at a faster rate for several hours afterward. Since exercise and physical activity burn calories and increase your metabolism, you can increase calorie loss by more activity and more exercise.

Ways to Increase Your Metabolism

+ Don't skip breakfast.
+ Don't skip any meal.
+ Eat smaller portions but eat more frequently (graze).
+ Don't stuff yourself.
+ Decrease stress any way you can.
+ Never go hungry.
+ Increase physical activity any way you can.

Don't Do What Sumo Wrestlers Do!

Sumo wrestlers are, by far, the world's authority when it comes to enhancing weight gain. In fact, they are constantly trying to increase their weight and body fat as much as possible. For a sumo wrestler, the extra weight is crucial to success. The heavier sumo wrestler has an edge over the lighter competitor.

Sumo wrestlers are allowed to eat a maximum of twice a day—preferably one gigantic meal—and, as a rule, they have to skip breakfast. Intuitively, you would think that they would be eating all day long to gain all that body weight. But for centuries, sumo wrestlers have been taught that they should eat one gigantic meal and then nap afterward. This gigantic meal is the equivalent of five to seven meals for the average person.

There is an important, logical reason for this practice. Research indicates that skipping a meal and then consuming a big meal can make you fat (184). This practice will make you prone to weight gain in the form of fat, compared to eating five or six small meals a day (grazing). Though the traditional sumo wrestling practices for gaining weight are the result of many years of experience, it is not clear if the sumo trainers knew that this practice of skipping breakfast promoted weight gain. One thing is evident: people who skip breakfast lose control of their appetite at lunch. Skipping breakfast is one characteristic that is very common to overweight and obese people. By skipping a meal, you will compensate with the next meal. In addition, it has been shown that skipping breakfast can reduce your metabolic rate by 5 percent.

So, don't skip any meal, especially breakfast.

Don't Do What Sumo Wrestlers Do

+ What sumo wrestlers do:
    + skip breakfast
    + eat one or two large meals
    + nap after meals
    + drink large amounts of beer
    + eat large/gigantic portions
+ What you should do:
    + eat breakfast
    + eat many times a day, smaller portions
    + don't sleep right after you eat
    + don't drink too much beer

Eat More Low-Glycemicx Index Foods—50 or Below

Low-Glycemic Index foods are generally high in fiber content. Think "unprocessed."

Low-Glycemic Index foods help maintain steady blood-sugar levels, thereby reducing appetite fluctuations and food cravings. This can be especially beneficial to people with diabetes. Foods low on the Glycemic Index will also help regulate your appetite and suppress your hunger. In addition, they will make you feel full for longer periods.

However, keep in mind that even if a food has a low Glycemic Index rating, it doesn't mean it is low in calories or even nutritious.

How to Use the Glycemic Index

There are a couple of different indexes available. One uses white bread as a standard, with the white bread rated as 100. However, most Glycemic Index tables use glucose, with a rating of 100, as the standard.

Glycemic Index Table

All Bran with Fiber 38	All-Bran 42
Apple 40	Apple juice 58
Apple juice, unsweetened 40	Apricots, canned 64
Apricots, canned syrup 91	Apricots, dried 30
Apricots, fresh 57	Artichoke 15
Asparagus 15	Baby lima beans, frozen 32
Bagel, white 103	Baked Beans 48
Banana 52	Banana bread 47
Barley, cracked 72	Barley, pearled 36
Barley, rolled 94	Basmati rice 58,
Beets 64	Black bean soup 92
Black beans, canned 69	Black-eyed peas 59
Black-eyed peas, canned 42	Blueberry muffin 59
Bran Buds 47	Bran Chex 58
Bran Flakes 74	Bran muffin 60
Broccoli 10	Buckwheat 54

Bulgur 48	Cabbage 10
Canned baked beans 48	Canned chickpeas 42
Canned kidney beans 52	Canned lentil soup 44
Canned peaches, natural juice 30	Canned pinto beans 45
Cantaloupe 65	Capellini 64
Carrot muffin 62	Carrots 49
Carrots, cooked 39	Cauliflower 15
Celery 15	Cheerios 106
Cheese tortellini 50	Cherries 22
Chickpeas, canned 42	Chickpeas, dried 28
Chocolate 70	Corn Bran 107
Corn Chex 83	Corn chips 105
Corn Flakes 92	Corn, fresh 60
Cornflakes 119	Cornmeal 98
Couscous 93	Cranberry juice 68
Cream of Wheat 66	Cream of Wheat Instant 74
Croissant 67	Cucumber 15
Custard 43	Dates 103
Doughnut 76	Dried apricots 31
Eggplant 15	Fat-free milk 32
Fettuccine 32	Fettuccine (egg) 32
Figs, dried 61	French baguette 95
French Fries 75	Fructose 32
Fruit Cocktail 55	Garbanzo beans 47
Glucose 137	Gnocchi 95
Golden Grahams 102	Graham Wafers 106
Granola Bars 61	Grapefruit 25
Grapefruit juice 48	Grapenuts 71
Grapes 43	Green beans 15
Green peas 48	Green pea soup, canned 94
Hamburger bun 87	High-fiber rye crispbread 93
High-fructose corn syrup 89	Honey 83
Ice cream 87	Ice cream, low-fat 71
Instant noodles 67	Jelly beans 114

Kaiser rolls 104	Kellogg's All Bran Fruit 'n Oats 55
Kellogg's Honey Smacks 78	Kellogg's Just Right 84
Kellogg's Mini-Wheats 81	Kidney beans 42
Kidney beans, canned 52	Kidney beans, dried 28
Kiwifruit 52	Lactose 65
Lentil soup, canned 63	Lentils 29
Lettuce 10	Lettuce, all varieties 15
Life cereal 94	Life Saver 100
Lima beans 32	Linguine 46
Long-grain rice 47	Low-fat yogurt, <15
Low-fat yogurt, sugar sweetened 33	Macaroni 45
Macaroni and cheese 92	Mango 51
Mars Bar 91	Mars Chocolate 63
Mars Peanut M&Ms 46	Mars Skittles 98
Mars Snickers Bar 57	Mars Twix Cookie Bars 62
Milk chocolate 34	Milk, whole 39
Milk, skim 46	Millet 101
Mixed-grain bread 69	Mushrooms 10
Nutri-grain 94	Oat Bran 55
Oat-bran bread 48	Oatmeal, instant 49
Old-fashioned oatmeal 49	Onions 10
Orange 43	Orange juice, frozen or in carton 74
Orange juice, fresh 52	Papaya 56
Parboiled rice 47	Parsnips 97
Peach, canned 67	Peach, canned in juice 38
Peach, fresh 42	Peanuts 15
Pear, canned 63	Pear, fresh 38
Pearled barley 25	Peas, dried 22
Peas, green 38	Peppers, all varieties 15
Pineapple 46	Pineapple juice 46
Pinto beans 55	Pinto beans, canned 64
Pita bread, white 82	Pita, whole wheat 57
Plum 24	Popcorn 79
Post Flakes 114	Potato crisps 77

Potato, baked 121	Potato, instant 118
Potato, mashed 100	Potato, microwaved 117
Potato, white, boiled 80	Pretzels 116
Potato, red-skinned, boiled 88	Prunes 29
Puffed Wheat 67	Pumpernickel 41
Pumpkin 75	Quick oats 66
Raisin Bran 61	Raisins 56
Ravioli, meat filled 56	Red Peppers 10
Rice bran 27	Rice cakes 82
Rice Chex 127	Rice crackers 91
Rice Krispies 82	Rice vermicelli 58
Rice, brown 79	Rice, instant, boiled 65
Rice, white 83	Rich Tea cookies 79
Rutabaga 103	Rye bread 48
Scones 92	Shortbread 91
Shredded Wheat 75	Snow peas 15
Sourdough 53	Soy beans 25
Soy milk 30	Spaghetti 41
Spaghetti, protein enriched 38	Spaghetti, white 38
Spinach 15	Spirali 61
Split pea soup 89	Sponge cake 46
Squash 15	Stone-ground whole wheat 53
Stoned Wheat Thins 96	Strawberries 40
Sucrose 92	Sweet corn 55
Sweet potato 54	Taco shell 68
Tapioca, boiled with milk 115	Tomato soup 38
Tomatoes 15	Tortellini, cheese 71
Vanilla wafers 110	Water crackers 102
Watermelon 72	Wheat bread, 112
Wheat bread, gluten free 129	Wheat crackers 96
Wheat kernels 59	Cream of Wheat, quick cooking 77
White potato 56	White rice 72,
White-skinned mashed potato 70	Whole Meal Rye 58
Whole milk 31	Whole wheat 77

Whole-wheat spaghetti 37	Yam 37
Yellow split peas 32	Yogurt, artificially sweetened 14
Yogurt, low fat, plain 20	Yogurt, low fat, fruit 47
Yogurt, sweetened 33	Zucchini 15

Summary

Eliminate bad calories from high-Glycemic Index carbohydrates. This group includes processed carbohydrates—especially sugar and white flour—and all foods made from these ingredients. Also, eliminate foods like corn syrup, molasses, honey, soft drinks, and beer.

Increase good calories, which are from low-Glycemic Index carbohydrates. This group includes high-fiber vegetables and fruits, and lean meats. Restrict your calorie intake and increase your physical activity to increase your metabolism.

Chapter Four

O of L.O.V.E.

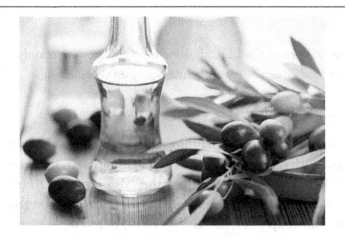

Oils: Olive Oil and Its Equivalent: Not All Fats Are Bad for You!

Fat is an essential nutrient that maintains the integrity of the cell membranes in the body. It is also needed to (1) help the body absorb fat-soluble vitamins, such as vitamins A, D, E, and K, and (2) provide a concentrated source of energy that is stored in fat cells for future use. Many health professionals, including nutritionists, recommend a consumption of no more than 30 percent of daily calories from fat. Of course, all fats are not the same. Most fat consumption should be from healthier, unsaturated fats.

Fat Intake

Of the recommended maximum 30 percent of calories per day from fat, less than 10 percent should come from saturated fat (such as fat from meat, butter, and eggs). In addition, you should limit the amount of cholesterol in your diet. Your diet should include no more than three hundred milligrams of cholesterol per day.

Saturated Fats: The Bad Cholesterol Maker

Saturated fats are found chiefly in beef and dairy products. A high intake of saturated fats tends to raise bad cholesterol—LDL—levels. LDL cholesterol is associated with an increased risk of heart disease. Intake of saturated fatty acids is directly related to increased risk factors for several diseases, including heart disease, stroke, breast cancer, prostate cancer, small intestine cancer, and overall mortality (185–195).

Trans Fats: The Bad Cholesterol Maker

Trans fats also raise the LDL cholesterol level. They are mainly found in processed foods that use partially hydrogenated vegetable oils.

Polyunsaturated Fats: The Good Cholesterol Maker

Polyunsaturated fats are the healthier fats. The human body cannot make these fats, which are needed by cells. Polyunsaturated fats have been shown to lower LDL cholesterol levels, but they also lower HDL (the good) cholesterol. Polyunsaturated fats are found in some nuts and vegetable oils, and should make up 10 percent or less of daily calories.

Monounsaturated Fats: The Good Cholesterol Maker

Monounsaturated fats are found in most nuts and olive oil. These fats have been shown to lower total cholesterol and LDL cholesterol levels, while maintaining the beneficial HDL cholesterol level associated with lowering the risk of heart disease. Up to 20 percent of daily calories should come from monounsaturated fat.

Oils

In spite of all the anxiety about fat in our diet, the body does require fat to function. The trouble is that most people eat the wrong kinds of fats and are lacking the good fats. Your body cannot function well without the two important polyunsaturated fats: linoleic and alpha-linolenic acids. These fatty acids are essential to normal cell structure and body function.

Both high- and low-fat diets can be bad for your health. The important goal should be to avoid the bad oils, and eat the good ones. Generally speaking, unextracted oils are better than chemically extracted ones, and unrefined ones are better than refined, because minimally processed oils tend to be high in antioxidants. The reason for this difference is that the modern way of processing of processing plant, nuts, and vegetable oils is by chemical extraction, using solvent extracts. This chemical extraction is preferred by the commercial factories, since it produces higher yields and is also quicker and less expensive (196). The most common solvent is petroleum-derived hexane . This technique is used for most of the "newer" industrial oils, such as soybean and corn oils. Therefore, by far, the best oil is extra virgin, cold-pressed olive oil.

Monounsaturated oils are good because they lower only LDL cholesterol. However, the ratio of the monounsaturated to saturated fat appears more important than total fat consumed. It's not so important to take in a great amount of monounsaturated fats, but it is important that your monounsaturated fats outnumber your saturated ones. Polyunsaturated oils are a mix of good and bad oils. However, certain polyunsaturated oils are important: the essential fatty acids omega-3 and omega-6.

In summary, most of your oil intake should come from food, not from extracted oil in a bottle. When you do use oil in a bottle, go for the unrefined. Rigorously limit trans fats and saturated fats. Limit polyunsaturated fats except for sources high in omega-3.

It is well known that saturated fats from animal products contribute to many diseases. Many researchers believe that the fats in Western diets are contributing to an increase in inflammatory and autoimmune diseases. Statistically, we consume too many of the bad fats, which promote inflammation, and not enough of the good fats, which produce the chemicals to counter it.

Tropical oils refer to oils made from palm, palm kernel, and coconut oils. These oils are used mostly in foods for several reasons. Firstly, they are excellent for shortening, because they don't get rancid easily. Secondly, they produce flaky pastry and appetizing color on fried foods. Thirdly, they don't give a greasy feel to foods like crackers. Due to these characteristics, it is difficult to substitute other vegetable oils for the tropical ones, since their polyunsaturated fats have a short shelf life.

Tropical oils, like palm oil, coconut oil, and rice bran oil, are particularly valued in Asian cultures for high-temperature cooking, because of their unusually high flash point.

The Bad Fats/Oils	
Saturated fats	Raise overall cholesterol Raise LDL cholesterol
Trans fats	Raise LDL cholesterol Lower HDL cholesterol
The Good Fats/Oils	
Monounsaturated fats	Lower cholesterol Lower LDL cholesterol Increase the HDL cholesterol
Polyunsaturated fats	Lower cholesterol Lower LDL cholesterol

Nuts Are Packed with Nutrition

Even though nuts are full of energy, some studies have shown that people who consume more nuts have a lower BMI (197–199). Nuts can help you with weight control. Use nuts as between-meal snacks; they have rich flavors and are quite satisfying.

Nuts are also full of vitamins and minerals. They contain many macronutrients and micronutrients, including fiber, protein, carbohydrates, fat (good oil), vitamin E, calcium, magnesium, and potassium. In addition, nuts also contain a wide variety of phytochemicals— such as phytosterols (beta-sitosterol), carotenoids, flavonoids, and proanthocyanidins—which may help protect against heart disease, cancer, and other chronic diseases.

Nuts

Nuts are a combination of the seed and the fruit, where the fruit does not open to release the seed. According to culinary definition, any large, oily kernel found within a shell and used in food may be regarded as a nut. This is a much less restrictive definition than used in botany. From a culinary point of view, many seeds are called nuts when they are not. Peanuts are actually legumes. Cashews are a "false fruit" that forms off the end of the cashew flower. Many other "nuts," such as almonds, pistachios, and coconuts, are actually drupes. Drupes occur when a fleshy outside layer surrounds a hard-walled seed, such as a peach. Pine nuts are coniferous seeds. Macadamias are kernels of seeds (200–202).

Because nuts generally have high oil content, they are a highly prized food and energy source. Many different seeds are edible by humans and can be eaten raw, used in cooking, or roasted as a snack food. In addition, they can be pressed for oil that is used in cooking and cosmetics.

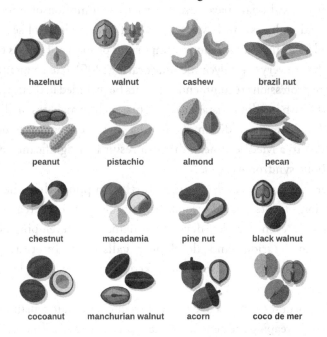

hazelnut	walnut	cashew	brazil nut
peanut	pistachio	almond	pecan
chestnut	macadamia	pine nut	black walnut
cocoanut	manchurian walnut	acorn	coco de mer

Nuts contain high concentrations of linoleic and linolenic acids, the vital fatty acids critical for growth, physical and mental development, optimal immunological responses, and blood clotting. It is important to note that since the oil/fat in nuts are mainly unsaturated fats, most specifically monounsaturated fats, their consumption does not elevate blood cholesterol. Furthermore, nuts contain many important nutrients such as:

+ Natural vitamins (vitamins E, folic acid, and B2)
+ Fiber

- Protein

- Essential minerals, such as magnesium, phosphorus, copper, and selenium

Consumption of nuts was first linked to protection against coronary disease in the early 1990s. Several epidemiological studies have since demonstrated a strong link between regular consumption of nuts and decreased risk of coronary disease (203–207). Four other large studies have confirmed the benefits to the heart of eating nuts (208–212).

Other clinical trials have revealed that consumption of nuts such as almonds and walnuts can lower the level of bad cholesterol-serum LDL cholesterol concentrations. Another important property of nuts is that they generally have a very low Glycemic Index rating (205). Consequently, many health-care professions recommend that nuts be included in diets prescribed for patients with insulin resistance problems, such as diabetes mellitus type II (206). For example, addition of a regular intake of about two ounces of nuts per day to a Mediterranean diet can result in a significant reversal of the metabolic syndrome (207).

Other clinical research findings further support that the regular consumption of nuts has additional benefits related to decreased risk of cardiovascular event, stroke, developing dementia, developing advanced macular degeneration, and developing gallstones. Interestingly, the consumption of nuts has also been linked to an increase in longevity of approximately two years (206).

It is important to emphasize that the frequency of nut consumption is a major factor in reaping the benefits of these precious foods. That is, the more often you consume nuts, the more you benefit from their health effects. For example, the risk of fatal coronary disease and the risk of developing type II diabetes both appear to decrease in linear fashion as nut consumption increases from less than once a week to daily (212, 213).

Besides the definite advantage of eating nuts for cardiovascular health, as well as protection against the development of type II diabetes, research has shown their benefit against the development of prostate cancer (214–221).

Clinical research trials on consumption of almonds, walnuts, peanuts, hazelnuts, pecans, macadamias, and pistachios show significant decreases in both total and LDL cholesterol levels.

One ounce of most nuts contains one hundred fifty to two hundred calories, with fifteen to twenty grams of fat. Even though nuts are high in fat and calories, they are full of important nutrients. Nuts are a significant source of protein. They're also rich in important minerals, such as copper, magnesium, zinc, iron, and calcium. In addition, nuts are good sources of fiber. But the good benefits do not stop there. Nuts are full of antioxidants and phytochemicals. Antioxidants fight against heart disease and certain kinds of cancer. Phytochemicals (flavonoids, indoles, phenolic acid, and plant sterols) reduce the risk of a number of chronic diseases, including cancer and heart disease. As with all foods, the key is moderation. In a July 2003 ruling, the Food and Drug Administration granted processors of certain nuts the right to print this statement on their labels: "Scientific evidence suggests but does not prove that eating 1.5 ounces per day of most nuts as part of a diet low in saturated fat and cholesterol may reduce the risk of heart disease." Remember, one and one-half ounces of nuts is about a handful, or one-third cup.

Most of the fats in nuts are unsaturated and are naturally cholesterol free. Nuts also contain vitamin E, folic acid, and plant fiber, which can reduce cholesterol levels. In addition, nuts contain arginine, which is a precursor to nitric acid, a substance that relaxes the blood vessels and prevents clotting. Certain nuts, such as walnuts, contain alpha-linolenic acid, which is a precursor of omega-3 fatty acid, which protects against heart disease.

Omega-3 and Omega-6 Essential Fatty Acids

Omega-3 and omega-6 fatty acids belong to a family of fats called essential fatty acids (EFA). These essential fatty acids are found in polyunsaturated fats. In the body, alpha-linolenic acid, an omega-3 fatty acid, is in shortest supply. You have to eat at least two servings of fatty fish per week to take in the required amount. In addition, you should include vegetable oils such as soybean oil, canola oil, and flaxseed oil, as well as nuts and seeds such as walnuts and flaxseeds in your diet. These oils and food sources are high in alpha-linolenic acid, which is essential for a healthy diet.

Vegetable oils and fats are derived from plants. Even though these oils are liquid at room temperature, the fats are solid. Both vegetable oils and fats are composed of triglycerides and varying blend of fatty acids (free fatty acids, monoglycerides, and diglycerides). A major portion of vegetable oil in commercial use is extracted from plant seeds. It should be emphasized that not all kinds of vegetable fats and oils may be edible. For example, processed linseed oil, tung oil, and castor oil used in lubricants, paints, cosmetics, pharmaceuticals, and other industrial purposes, are inedible.

Plant-Derived Oils

- palm
- soybean
- rapeseed
- sunflower seed peanut
- cottonseed
- palm kernel
- coconut
- olive
- grapeseed oil
- sesame seed oil
- Wheat Germ Oil

Extraction

Nowadays, the extraction of vegetable oils is done chemically. In this technique, solvent extracts, which are commonly petroleum-based, are used to get a higher yield more quickly and inexpensively. This chemical extraction is used for most of the commercially used oils, such as soybean and corn oils.

A healthier technique is the traditional physical extraction, which does not use any form of solvent. This method is commonly used to produce the more traditional oils, like olive oil. It is important to emphasize that this physical extraction is preferred by most health-care providers and dietitians, not to mention customers interested in healthier foods.

In the processing of edible oils, the oil is heated under a vacuum to near the smoking point, and water is introduced at the bottom of the oil. The water is immediately converted to steam, which bubbles through the oil, carrying with it any chemicals that are water soluble. This process is called sparging. The sparging removes impurities that can impart unwanted flavors and odors into the oil.

The American diet has a high range of omega-6 fatty acids. The ration is between 10- and 20-to-1 in favor of omega 6, which is not good for your health. You should increase your intake of omega-3 fatty acids and reduce your intake of omega-6 fatty acids. Omega-6 and omega-3 EFAs are best consumed in a ratio of about 3:1, that is three portions of omega-6 for each portion of omega-3 fatty acid. Sources of omega-3 fatty acids include flaxseed oil (the richest natural source), flax seeds, rapeseed oil, pumpkin seeds, soybean oil, walnut oil, walnuts, and oily fish.

Table 3. Omega-3 and Omega-6 Fatty Acid Contents of Some Seeds (gram/100 grams)

Omega-3 Fatty Acid (100g)	(g)	Omega-6 Fatty Acid (100g)	(g)
Flaxseeds	20	Flaxseeds	6
Pumpkin seeds	10	Pumpkin seeds	20
Sunflower seeds	Trace	Sunflower seeds	30
Sesame seeds	Trace	Sesame seeds	25
Pine nuts	1	Pine nuts	25

Table 4. Omega-3 and Omega-6 Fatty Acid Contents of Some Seed Oils (gram/100 gram)

Omega-3 Fatty Acid (100g)	(g)	Omega-6 Fatty Acid (100g)	(g)
Flaxseed oil	58	Safflower oil	74
Flaxseed oil	30	Grapeseed oil	68
Walnut oil	12	Sunflower oil	63
Canola oil	7	Walnut oil	58
Soybean oil	7	Soybean oil	51
Wheat germ oil	5	Corn oil	50

Table 5. Omega-3 and Omega-6 Fatty Acid Contents of Nuts (gram/100 grams)

Omega-3 Fatty Acid (100g)	(g)	Omega-6 Fatty Acid (100g)	(g)
Walnuts	5.5	Walnuts	28
Hazelnuts	Trace	Hazelnuts	4
Cashews	Trace	Cashews	8
Almonds	Trace	Almonds	10
Brazils	Trace	Brazils	23

Benefits of Some Good Oils

Sesame Oil

+ Contains vitamin E
+ Contains vitamin B6

Walnut Oil

+ Reduces heart disease
+ Lowers triglycerides

Peanut Oil

+ Reduces heart disease
+ Contains resveratrol, the substance in grapes and red wine
+ Reduces cardiovascular disease
+ Reduces cancer risk

Grapeseed Oil

+ Reduces LDL cholesterol
+ Reduces heart disease
+ Increases HDL cholesterol

Flaxseed Oil

- Lowers cholesterol
- Thins blood
- Reduces inflammation
- Improves kidney function

Olive Oil

- Full of antioxidants
- Lowers LDL
- Raises HDL
- Protects blood vessels
- Promotes healthy skin

Almond Oil

- Reduces the risk of certain diseases, such as gallstones, type I diabetes, colon cancer, heart disease
- Reduces blood pressure
- Reduces atherosclerosis by lowering cholesterol
- Aids in weight loss
- Contains the anti-cancer agent laetril

Good Cooking Oils

- Canola Oil
- Corn Oil
- Flaxseed Oil
- Peanut Oil
- Olive Oil
- Safflower Oil
- Sunflower Oil

Bad Cooking Oils

- Butter
- Coconut Oil
- Margarine
- Palm Oil
- Palm Kernel Oil
- Vegetable Shortening
- Lard

The table shows, in grams, how much saturated, monounsaturated, polyunsaturated trans. fats are contained in 100g of various commonly used oils and fats.

Oil	Total	Sat.	Poly.	Mono.
Canola	14	1	4	8
Corn	14	2	8	4
Flaxseed	14	1	10	3
Olive	14	2	1	10
Peanut	14	3	5	6
Safflower	14	2	10	2
Sesame	14	2	6	5
Sunflower seed	14	2	9	3

The table shows, in grams, how much saturated, monounsaturated, polyunsaturated trans. fats are contained in 100g of various commonly used seed/nut oils and fats.

Nuts	Total	Sat.	Poly.	Mono
Almond	14	1	3	10
Brazil	19	5	7	7
Cashew	13	2	8	3
Hazelnut	18	1	2	15
Macadamia	20	2	3	15
Pecan	19	2	5	12

Pistachio	14	2	4	8
Walnut	15	2	11	2

Fish	Omega-3
Cod	3.0
Flounder	0.2
Mackerel	1.8
Rockfish	0.8
Salmon	1.9
Sole (lemon)	0.2
Trout (rainbow)	0.5
Tuna, albacore	1.5
Tuna, blue fin	1.0

Comprehensive List of Vegetable Oils

+ Almond Oil
+ Apricot Kernel Oil
+ Avocado Oil
+ Canola Oil
+ Chile Oil
+ Coconut Oil
+ Cottonseed Oil
+ Flaxseed Oil
+ Grapeseed Oil
+ Hazelnut Oil
+ Macadamia Oil
+ Mustard Oil
+ Palm Oil
+ Palm Kernel Oil
+ Peanut Oil
+ Pine Seed Oil
+ Poppy Seed Oil
+ Pumpkin Seed Oil
+ Rice Bran Oil

- Safflower Oil
- Sesame Seed Oil
- Soybean Oil
- Sunflower Seed Oil
- Tea Oil
- Truffle Oil
- Walnut Oil
- Wheat Germ Oil

*Grams of Protein, Fat, Carbohydrates, and
Total Calories per Ounce of Nut*

Nut	Protein	Fat	Carbohydrates	Calories
Almonds	15	8	2.9	90
Beechnuts	1.8	1	3	6
Brazil Nuts	.1	4	1	97
Butternuts	5	2	1	20
Cashews	5	12	11	145
Chestnuts	6	.8	12	58
Coconut	1	7	10	106
Filberts	4	20	4	182
Ginkgo Nuts	1	4	21	90
Hazelnuts	4	20	4	182
Macadamia Nuts	1	23	3	218
Peanuts	9	14	8	152
Pecans	2	22	4	208
Pine Nuts	3	18	5	176
Pistachios	2	16	5	246
Walnuts	3	17	5	94
Walnuts (white)	5	5	14	196
Water Chestnut	1	7	6	97

Chapter Five

V of L.O.V.E.

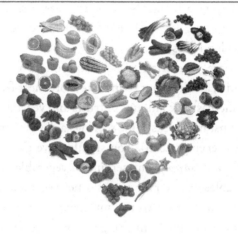

Vegetables, Fruits, and Herbs

Vegetables and Fruits

Fruits and vegetables are undoubtedly the most important part of any good diet. Almost everyone can benefit from eating more of them. Since no single fruit or vegetable provides all of the nutrients you need to be healthy, variety is as important as quantity. Therefore, success lies in the variety of different fruits and vegetables that you eat.

Research has shown that following a well-balanced, low-fat, high-fiber, vegetarian diet lowers the incidence of coronary artery disease, hypertension, obesity, and some forms of cancer (222–224). But you don't have to be a fruitarian, vegan, or lacto-vegetarian to benefit from the fruit and vegetarian diet.

A typical vegetarian diet closely matches expert dietary recommendations for healthy eating: low in saturated fat and high in fiber, complex carbohydrates, and fresh fruit and vegetables. Complex carbohydrates are basically those foods that are not processed and are not refined, such as whole fruits, vegetables, wholegrain, oats, muesli, and brown rice. Complex carbohydrates (whole fruits and vegetables) are broken down by digestion into glucose more slowly than simple carbohydrates (fruit juice) and thus provide a gradual steady stream of energy throughout the day. As long as you eat a variety of foods, you will get all the nutrients you need. Fruits and vegetables are rich in essential vitamins and minerals, fiber, carbohydrates, and phytochemicals. They have been associated with many health benefits, including lowered risk for certain cancers, stroke, heart disease, and high blood pressure.

Whether you are vegetarian or not, experiment with a diet high in vegetables and fruits, and attempt to include more meat-free dishes in your diet. You should increase the amount of fruits and vegetables you eat every day. You should consume at least nine servings a day rather than the often-recommended five servings (225). You should have three to five servings of vegetables each day. Simply, one serving of vegetables is about one cup of raw leafy vegetables or one-half cup of other vegetables, cooked or raw. In addition, you should have two to four servings of fruit each day. One serving of fruit can be one medium orange, apple or banana or one-half cup of chopped, cooked, or canned fruit (better if not sweetened).

Choose a variety of fruits and vegetables. It's easy to get into a rut when it comes to the food you eat. Break out and try a wider variety, being sure to include dark green, leafy vegetables along with yellow, orange, and red fruits and vegetables.

Herbs

Herbs are the leaves of herbaceous plants. Spices come from the other parts of the plant, such as the bark, root, bud, or berry. Most herbs have one or two main applications, though they may have dozens of minor uses. Active constituents of the herb are particular groups of chemicals, such as terpenes, alkaloids, and flavonoids. Fragrant herbs frequently owe their action to the volatile oils that give them their fragrance. Bitter herbs owe their action to alkaloids, saponins, or flavonoids that contribute to their bitterness.

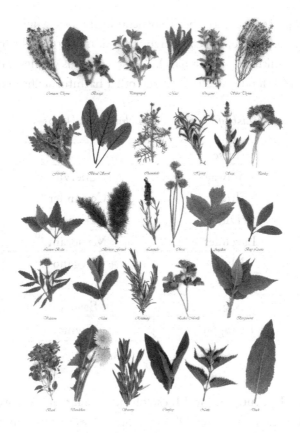

Herbs can provide good and essential nutrients, and their benefits are varied. Many herbs contain powerful ingredients and chemicals that can help your body heal and fight disease. Even today, herbs and spices are the primary source of health care for 80 percent of the world. Many herbs are rich in compounds that have a beneficial effect on certain tissues and organs and, therefore, can be used as medicines to treat, cure, or prevent disease. Compared to fruits and vegetables, herbs have a superior antioxidant activity. Some herbs suitable for instilling as teas are oregano, rosemary, peppermint, sage, spearmint, savory, and thyme, all of which have been shown to contain significant levels of antioxidants. The antioxidant activity of herbs is retained even after boiling for thirty minutes. However, it is recommended that you grind up dried herbs in a culinary mortar and pedestal for maximum flavor.

In general, fresh herbs and spices taste better and contain higher antioxidant levels compared to their processed counterparts. The antioxidant activity of culinary herbs and spices suggests that in addition to imparting flavor to food, they possess potential health benefits by inhibiting lipid peroxidation (oxidative degradation of lipids, whereby free radicals attack the lipids in cell membranes, resulting in cell damage). You should consider using more herbs for flavoring your food instead of salt and other harmful artificial chemicals.

A List of Common and Nutritious Herbs

Anise	Basil
Caraway	Chervil
Chives	Coriander
Dill	Fennel
Lavender	Marjoram
Mint	Oregano
Parsley	Rosemary
Sage	Savory
Tarragon	Thyme

DASH Diet

The National Institutes of Health established the famous and well-studied DASH diet, which stands for Dietary Approaches to Stop Hypertension, as a means of lowering blood pressure and cholesterol levels. This diet is recommended for everyone, especially people with high blood pressure. On the DASH diet, salt and sodium intake is restricted to achieve better control of blood pressure. It also emphasizes the importance of three minerals in controlling blood pressure: calcium, magnesium, and potassium. The DASH diet also greatly emphasizes the role of fruits and vegetables as well as low-fat dairy and meat products. Several studies have shown that the DASH diet lowers both systolic and diastolic blood pressure. Another important point is that this diet lowers blood pressure quickly—usually within two weeks!

The sodium recommendation in the original DASH diet is twenty-four hundred milligrams (one teaspoon of salt). A study called the DASH-sodium study showed even better blood pressure results with an intake of fifteen hundred milligrams daily.

Researchers have discovered that the additional fruits, vegetables, and whole grains that people consume while on the DASH diet provide a great deal of food compounds, such as lycopene, beta carotene, and isoflavones. These substances fall under the category of phytochemicals, substances plants naturally produce to protect themselves against harmful agents in nature, especially viruses, bacteria, and fungi. The class of phytochemicals include hundreds of naturally occurring substances, including carotenoids, flavonoids, indoles, isoflavones, capsaicin, and protease inhibitors. Even though the exact function of phytochemicals in promoting health is unclear, they may help protect against some cancers, heart disease, and other chronic health conditions, as they are scavengers of free radicals, harmful chemicals produced in the body.

The DASH diet naturally contains foods that produce a great deal of antioxidant activities and have the ability to lower blood homocysteine levels. High blood levels of this amino acid are associated with increased risk of cardiovascular disease. The DASH diet includes whole grains, poultry, fish, and nuts and reduced amounts of fats, red meat, sweets, and sugared beverages. In addition, the DASH diet advises consumption of low-fat and fat-free dairy foods.

Grains

Vegetables

Fruits

DASH Diet in Summary

8 servings

5 servings

5 servings

Low-fat fat or fat-free dairy Meats, poultry, and fish Nuts, seeds, and dry beans Fats and oils

Sweets

3 servings

2 servings

5 per week

3 per week

5 per week

A Balanced Diet Based on the DASH Diet

Use the most current food plate to maintain a healthy, balanced diet by eating foods from all the food groups. Each of these vegetarian food groups provides some, but not all, of the nutrients you need. Foods in one group can't replace those in another. No one food group is more important than another; for good health, you need them all.

Eggs: egg, egg whites, soy milk

Dairy: all types of cheese, yogurt, milk, cottage cheese

Nuts and Seeds: pine nuts, walnuts, pistachios, Brazil, pecans, almonds, sesame seeds, cashews, pumpkin seeds, hazelnuts, and macadamias

Oils: corn, canola, avocado, olive, soybean, safflower, peanut, and other nut and seed oils

Whole Grains: oats, wheat, rice, couscous, noodles, kasha, flax, bulgur, barley, whole-grain bread, rye, pita, tortilla, rice cakes, pasta, corn

Fruits and Vegetables: figs, grapes, raisins, pears, avocados, chiles, mushrooms, herbs, tomatoes, kale, oranges, broccoli, collards, kiwifruit, melons, chard, spices, okra, apples, sweet potatoes, bananas, peppers, asparagus, cucumbers, manioc, potatoes, lemon grasss, plum, cassavas, onions, cherries, guavas, carrots, cabbages, squash, leeks, eggplants, celery, and all kinds of legumes: soybeans, peanuts, red beans, lentils, peas, kidney beans, tofu, pea, dried peas, soy flour, chick peas, all kinds of beans

As part of the DASH diet regimen, animal protein intake should be limited to lean meat and poultry in moderate amounts one to three times per week. However, you should add fish and seafood to your diet, and consume them two to four times per week.

In summary, under the DASH diet, eat an abundance of vegetables, fruits, grains, beans, nuts, and seeds. Eat fresh and minimally processed food wherever possible. Increase intake of seasonally fresh and locally grown foods. Decrease your salt intake. Have a moderate intake of meat and poultry, but a relatively higher intake of fish and seafood.

How Many Servings of Fruits and Vegetables Should You Eat?

Current guidelines recommend *at least* two to four servings of fresh or dried fruits and three to five servings of cooked or uncooked vegetables each day (225).

What counts as a serving? One medium (regular size, or about three inches in diameter) apple or orange or banana equals a fruit serving, while half a cup of chopped vegetables is a vegetable serving.

Good Nutrients in Fruits and Vegetables

+ Vitamins—folate lowers levels of a heart-disease-promoting agent called homocysteine.

+ Minerals—potassium can help control blood pressure.

+ Flavonoids—plant chemicals act like antioxidants.

+ Phenols—organic compounds in foods act like antioxidants.

+ Carotenoids—contains compounds similar to vitamin A.

+ Fiber—can reduce the risk of blood clots.

Special Consideration for Vegans

Vegans should pay special attention to their vitamin B12 and vitamin D intake by eating fortified foods or taking vitamin B12/vitamin D supplements. Vitamin B12 is a member of the vitamin B complex. It contains cobalt and is also known as cobalamin.

Vitamin B12 is necessary for the synthesis of red blood cells, the maintenance of the nervous system, and growth and development in children. Deficiency can cause anemia. Vitamin B12 neuropathy, which involves the degeneration of nerve fibers and irreversible neurological damage, can also occur.

Vitamin B12 is exclusively synthesized by bacteria and found primarily in animal products such as meat, eggs, and dairy products. This essential vitamin cannot be made in significant quantity by plants and plant cells. Therefore, the present consensus is that any B12 present in plant foods is likely to be unavailable to humans, so these foods should not be relied on as safe sources. Currently, there are many vegan foods available on the market that are fortified with B12. They include nondairy milks, meat substitutes, breakfast cereals, and one type of nutritional yeast. High heat generated from cooking may destroy the B12 found naturally in animal foods. Cyanocobalmin, the form in fortified foods, may be more stable during cooking. For example, in an acid medium (pH 4–7), cyanocobalmin can withstand boiling at 120° C (226–235).

Chapter Six

E of L.O.V.E.

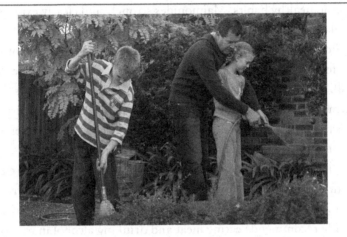

Exercise, Sexercise (Lovemaking)

The Bible and Maimonides on healthy body and physical activity

> Any person who increases his physical activity and exerts himself a lot, takes care not to eat to the point of being completely full, and keeps his bowels soft, illness will not come upon him and his strength will increase.

The Laws of Temperaments (Hilchot Deot) 4:15

According to the commandment in the Bible, "Only take heed to thyself, and keep thy soul diligently and safeguard your souls" (Deuteronomy 4:9), each person is obligated to safeguard his/her physical health. The commandment of safeguarding one's health is not only good advice, but also is an essential and fundamental law in the attainment of spirituality.

According to one of the prominent and exalted sages of the Bible, Rambam or better known as Maimonides (1135–1204 CE), this commandment teaches the importance and obligation of vigorous physical health. Besides being one of the greatest rabbinical scholars, an outstanding philosopher and a well-known physician of his time, Maimonides also served as the personal physician to the sultan of Egypt. Maimonides emphasized that physical health is an essential requirement for spiritual accomplishment.

In one of his greatest works, *Hilchot Deot (The Laws of Temperaments)*, he teaches ways to attain and enhance one's physical health. He holds that a person must distance himself from things that destroy the body and develop healthy habits. Maimonides strongly and clearly expresses the sacred relationship between mind-body-spiritual health.

He holds that maintaining a healthy physical body is vital for service of God, for one cannot understand or have any knowledge of the Creator if he is ill. Therefore, one must avoid and stay away from elements and acts that harm the body. One should diligently accustom oneself to routines and practices that are healthy and promote a healthy body. Maimonides devotes a substantial portion of his book to proper eating habits.

He enumerates in his book the beneficial as well as the harmful elements in human nutrition. He promotes a diet rich in vegetables and fruits like figs, pears, pomegranates, quinces, apples, melons, and different kinds of squash. He recommends eating meat and drinking alcohol in moderation. He states that by following this regimen, one will have more energy, greater concentration, and increased enthusiasm in all pursuits.

It is very interesting that this great sage comments on the importance of exercise and physical activity in *The Laws of Temperaments* (4:14) to physical health. Maimonides is keen on physical activity and regular exercise. He also stresses the fact that one should eat to keep the body healthy and not just to satisfy the palate; eat only when hungry, and stop eating before you fill up.

To support his teachings, Maimonides quotes King Solomon in Proverbs 13:25, that the righteous eats only to satiate his body and soul. Sages have interpreted this to mean that one has to eat for the health of the body that contains the soul. Indeed, all of us eat more than what we need. Moderation is almost completely forgotten by our society and unknown by the majority of us.

The first wealth is health.

Ralph Waldo Emerson

Physical Activity

Physical inactivity or lack of exercise is a major risk factor for developing coronary artery disease, obesity, high blood pressure, a low level of HDL, and diabetes. Therefore, ordinary physical activity and exercise are critically important for maintaining your optimal health, because they have many beneficial effects on most organ systems of your body. Additionally, regular physical activity has been shown to reduce the risks of developing many chronic diseases as well as reducing the chances of dying from them (236–251).

Medical research has demonstrated that nearly all individuals can benefit from regular physical activity. Therefore, physical fitness should be a priority for people of all ages.

Benefits of Regular Physical Activity and Exercise:

+ Reduces the risk of heart disease and other conditions
+ Reduces the risk of developing diabetes
+ Reduces the risk of developing high blood pressure
+ Reduces the level of blood pressure in people with high blood pressure
+ Reduces the risk of developing colon cancer
+ Reduces the risk of breast cancer
+ Reduces the risk of obesity and overweight
+ Reduces the risk of weight gain
+ Reduces the risk of brittle bones and fractures by improving bone density
+ Reduces the risk of deconditioning of your muscles
+ Reduces the risk of depression and anxiety
+ Increases levels of HDL, or "good cholesterol"
+ Lowers high blood pressure
+ Helps burn fat
+ Controls blood-sugar levels in diabetics and pre-diabetics
+ Boosts the immune system

Important Facts About Physical Activity

Many people defer physical activity because they believe in a myth that only vigorous exercise or playing sports counts as healthy activity. In fact, substantial health benefits can be achieved from regular activity without the need for special equipment, sporting ability, or getting very hot and sweaty. Interestingly, even moderately intense physical activity such as brisk walking is beneficial. There is strong scientific evidence that supports the notion that moderately intense physical activity (see below) is enough to bring about real benefits in terms of promoting health and preventing illnesses (252). Regular activity can also improve the way you look and feel. In combination with a balanced diet, regular activity can help to maintain a healthy weight. It can even boost self-confidence and reduce the risk of depression.

Do Physical Activity to FIT

Any goal or plan designed to improve physical fitness takes into account three important factors: (1) frequency, (2) intensity, and (3) time—FIT. The FIT formula provides the best conditioning.

The FIT formula:

F = frequency (how often/days per week)

I = intensity (how hard/percentage of heart rate)

T = time (amount for each session or day)

What is most important is to attempt to include all sorts of physical activities in your daily life.

Recommendations for exercise or physical activity:

+ At least thirty minutes of moderate activity at least five days per week

+ At least twenty minutes of vigorous physical activity at least three times per week

Activities to FIT in your daily life routine:

Moderate activities

+ Walking for pleasure

+ Gardening and yard work

+ Brisk walking

+ Hiking

+ Housework, dancing

Vigorous activities

+ Stair climbing, aerobic exercise

+ Jogging, running

+ Bicycling, rowing, and swimming

+ Activities such as soccer and basketball that include continuous running

+ Tennis, racquetball, soccer, basketball, and touch football

Any Physical Activity Is a Form of Exercise

It is important to note that exercise is a form of physical activity. Are there any differences between exercise and routine physical activities of daily living? Simply put, both can burn calories. Physical activities are routine activities that you might perform daily, such as shopping, cleaning, gardening, and walking the dog. Exercise is a special form of physical activity that is specifically planned, structured, and repetitive in nature. That structure and repetitiveness are why some people find it difficult to stick to an exercise plan. Regularly doing the types of physical activities you enjoy can substitute for the unattractive, mechanical forms of exercise and improve your ability to do the everyday activities you enjoy.

The good news is that *every* type of activity burns calories, even sitting, breathing, chewing, and sleeping. The more vigorous, strenuous, and energetic an activity, the more calories are burned. But there are many ways to be do physical activities besides the "dreary" and "tedious" exercise such as stair climbing and treadmill. Find several different activities that you enjoy, and include them in your regular routine weekly activities. Consider doing more of the following physical activities that you might not have considered exercise but which will still be beneficial.

+ Walking up stairs instead of using elevators
+ Walking up moving escalators
+ For short distances, walking instead of driving
+ Doing the housework at a faster pace
+ Gardening or raking leaves
+ Dancing, singing, belly dancing

Understanding Weight-Loss Plateaus

It is an inevitable truth that almost everyone reaches a weight-loss plateau at some point in their diet. The reason underlying this "physiological plateau" is that the human body is extremely efficient and can adapt to many different extreme situations, including calorie restriction. The ultimate objective of the body is to keep energy intake and output in balance (see chapter 12).

L.O.V.E. Diet Gear
Anti-Plateau Gear

This patented and newly invented weight-loss gear is a uniquely designed bodysuit you can wear to battle the notorious plateau effect seen with many exercises. By wearing it, you can also increase you BMR and achieve a greater amount of calorie burning per unit of time.

However, the most important benefit of this special exercise gear is to fight and overcome one of the most dreadful points of any weight-loss program, the "plateau effect," which is seen with all types of weight-loss programs. As it was explained before, it is an inevitable truth that almost everyone reaches a weight-loss plateau at some point in their diet.

Lovemaking and Calories

Researchers have studied the effect of lovemaking on almost every part of the body, from the brain to the heart to the immune system. Studies confirm that an active sex life may lead to many health benefits (252–287).

These include a longer life, better cardiovascular health, improved ability to ward off pain, a more robust immune system, and even protection against certain cancers, not to mention lower rates of depression.

The Benefits of Lovemaking (Sex)

Lovemaking increases longevity

Lovemaking improves cardiovascular health

Lovemaking improves blood pressure control

Lovemaking lowers risk of breast cancer

Lovemaking lowers prostate cancer risk

Lovemaking relieves/reduces pain

Lovemaking increases muscle leanness/a slimmer physique

Lovemaking increases testosterone and estrogen levels

Lovemaking decreases symptoms of menopause

Lovemaking improves quality of semen

Lovemaking relieves stress

Lovemaking boosts immunity

Lovemaking burns calories

Lovemaking improves the sense of intimacy

Lovemaking strengthens pelvic floor muscles

Lovemaking improves sleep quality

Lovemaking promotes happiness and satisfaction

Lovemaking improves breathing

Lovemaking strengthens bones and muscles

Lovemaking reduces risk of prostate disease

Lovemaking lowers cholesterol

Lovemaking boosts level of immunoglobulin A, the antibody that fights off illness.

Sex Increases Longevity

Men (young or old) who have intercourse more often live longer, and women who reported enjoying sex more lived longer than those who didn't report enjoyment (253–260).

Sex Improves Cardiovascular Health

In a British study, the researchers found that having sex twice or more a week reduced the risk of fatal heart attack by half for the men, compared with those who had sex less than once a month (254–258).

Sex Improves Blood Pressure Control

In a study published in the journal *Biological Psychology,* people who had sex more often tended to have lower diastolic blood pressure, or the bottom number in a blood pressure reading (253–258, 261).

Sex Decreases Risk of Breast Cancer

A French study found that women who have vaginal intercourse not at all or infrequently had three times the risk of breast cancer, compared with women who had intercourse more often (255).

Sex Lowers Prostate Cancer Risk

Frequent ejaculations may reduce the risk of prostate cancer later in life, Australian researchers reported in the *British Journal of Urology International.* Another study, reported in the *Journal of the American Medical Association,* found that frequent ejaculations, twenty-one or more a month, were linked to lower prostate cancer risk in older men, compared to men with ejaculations of four to seven monthly. In another study, men who had intercourse more than three thousand times in their lives had half the prostate cancer risk of those who had not. It seems that men who have more intercourse tend to have better prostate function and eliminated more waste products in their semen (262–263).

Sex Relieves/Reduces Pain

Sex results in release of the hormone called oxytocin, which can lead to the release of endorphins, a potent pain reliever. In a study published in the *Bulletin of Experimental Biology and Medicine*, forty-eight volunteers who inhaled oxytocin vapor and then had their fingers pricked found their pain threshold lowered by more than half. Others have conducted studies suggesting that more sexual activity helps relieve lower back pain and migraines (253–257). So, if you are suffering from headaches, arthritis pain, or even PMS symptoms, they may improve after sexual intercourse.

Sex Increases Muscle Leanness/A Slimmer Physique

A study of healthy German adults revealed that men and women who had sex more frequently tended to be slimmer than folks who didn't have as much sex. Sex burns about sixty calories per encounter, therefore, having sex three times a week for a month would burn about seven hundred calories, or the equivalent of jogging about seven miles (252–256).

Sex Increases Testosterone and Estrogen Levels

A group of men being treated for erectile problems saw greater increases in testosterone levels when, along with the treatments, they had frequent sex. Specifically, men who had sex at least eight times per month had greater increases than those who had sex fewer than eight times per month (253–257).

Sex Decreases Symptoms of Menopause

Menopausal women in Nigeria experienced fewer hot flashes when they had sex more frequently. Brody says this may be because sexual activity helps regulate hormonal levels, which in turn affect the symptoms of menopause (253–255).

Sex Improves Quality of Semen

In three studies, men who had frequent intercourse had a higher volume of semen, a higher sperm count, and a higher percentage of healthier sperm, compared with men who tended to participate in other sexual activities (254–256).

Sex Relieves Stress

A big health benefit of sex is lower blood pressure and overall stress reduction, according to researchers from Scotland who reported their findings in the journal *Biological Psychology*. According to the findings of their research, those who had intercourse had better responses to stress than those who engaged in other sexual behaviors or abstained (254–258). Another study published in the same journal found that frequent intercourse was associated with lower diastolic blood pressure in cohabiting participants. Yet other research found a link between partner hugs and lower blood pressure in women.

Sex Boosts Immunity

Good sexual health may mean better physical health. Having sex once or twice a week has been linked with higher levels of an antibody called immunoglobulin A, or IgA, which can protect you from getting colds and other infections. Regular sex could help to ward off colds and flu. Psychologists in Pennsylvania have shown that people who have sex once or twice a week get a boost to their immune systems (254–258).

Sex Burns Calories

Sex is a great mode of exercise. It takes good amount of energy to perform it well. (See section on sexercise on page 000.)

Sex Improves the Sense of Intimacy

As a result of having sex and orgasms, the levels of the hormone oxytocin is increased. Besides being a pain reliever, oxytocin, the so-called love hormone, helps us bond and build trust. Researchers from the University of Pittsburgh and the University of North Carolina evaluated fifty-nine premenopausal women before and after warm contact with their husbands and partners ending with hugs. They found that the more contact, the higher the oxytocin levels. Oxytocin allows us to feel the urge to nurture and to bond and be more giving and generous (253–256).

Sex Strengthens Pelvic Floor Muscles

Women having sexual intercourse and performing pelvic floor muscle exercises (also known as Kegel) during sex will enjoy more pleasure, as well as strengthen the pelvic area. This ultimately helps to minimize the risk of stress and overflow incontinence later in life.

To perform the Kegel exercise, you must attempt to tighten the muscles of your pelvic floor. This exercise can be performed throughout the day in many different situations. Tighten your pelvic muscles as if you're trying to stop urine flow. Keep those muscles tightened for several seconds. Count to three and then release. Repeat this ten times.

Sex Improves Quality of Sleep

According to research studies, the oxytocin released during orgasm also promotes sleep (253–258, 484–487). Consequently, adequate sleep has been linked with maintaining a healthy weight and blood pressure.

Furthermore, lovemaking (sex) also promotes happiness and satisfaction, improves breathing, strengthens bones and muscles, lowers cholesterol, and boosts level of immunoglobulin A, the antibody that fights off illness and infections (266–287, 488–506).

In addition, enthusiastic and energetic intercourse and lovemaking can burn up calories at a fast rate. The calories burned during lovemaking can range between one hundred and four hundred an hour, depending on the intensity and the length of lovemaking (288–289).

We all want to look and feel sexier and more attractive to our mates. The emotional and psychological support of your mate or your loved one is a very important factor in weight loss and weight-control success.

Lovemaking as Sexercise

The feeling and expression of intimacy during lovemaking or sexual activity can make you feel great mentally and emotionally. There is plenty of evidence in the medical literature to support that the act of lovemaking has benefits for your physical, emotional, and psychological well-being.

The average number of calories you can burn during lovemaking varies, but lovemaking is equivalent to a workout, raising your heart rate and pumping oxygenated blood around the body to the vital organs, including your genitalia and erogenous zones. The number of calories burned during lovemaking as with other activities is a function of many different factors, including intensity, effort, frequency, your weight, ambient temperature, duration, and position.

Basically, lovemaking and sexual activity is a form of exercise, which is good for you, so lovemaking can be nicknamed Sexercise. Sexercise is a good exercise, which lowers your blood pressure, increases your muscle tone, and improves your cardiovascular health.

It is well known that lovemaking and exercise can reduce stress, so doing either one, or a combination of both, on a regular basis will destress you and keep you relaxed and, ultimately, happy.

Kissing

Kissing your lover can burn between one hundred fifty and three hundred calories an hour, or approximately three to five calories per minute. Therefore, every kiss counts. A really passionate kiss can burn up twelve calories, but on average, every kiss uses six calories. So, go on and kiss more, and kiss for longer.

Kissing is also great for your teeth and oral hygiene. The act of kissing increases saliva production, and saliva has an important role in preventing tooth decay. Saliva is nature's cleansing process, which washes out the mouth and helps remove the cavity-causing food particles that accumulate after meals. In addition, it washes away plaque from your teeth, and the minerals found in saliva help repair early tooth decay. Saliva also limits bacterial growth and neutralizes damaging acids in your mouth (286, 287, 481–483).

Foreplay

The longer the foreplay, the better the lovemaking and the more calories you will burn with each lovemaking session. It is estimated that you can burn between eighty to two hundred calories in thirty minutes of sexual intercourse. Naturally, this depends on the position you choose and how energetic your lovemaking is. Combination of foreplay and other forms of intimacy with intercourse can yield varying degrees of calorie burn (288, 289). The more intense the sex, the more calories are burned. Having an active sex life of three times a week burns fifteen thousand to seventy-five thousand calories per year. Each pound of fat contains thirty-five hundred calories. So, doing the simple math, in one year you can lose five to twenty pounds of fat with an active sex life!

You Can Improve Your Sex Life with Exercise

Exercise can help you get more satisfaction from sex. It can also increase your potency and improve your lovemaking. Studies have found a direct correlation between physical inactivity and a lack of potency. In other words, exercise can get you in shape and increase your potency, and it can also make your love life more enjoyable.

For an energetic sex life, and to get the most out of your sex life, you will need the following exercises:

+ Endurance exercises like repetitive lifting of light weights

+ Cardiovascular endurance exercises like running, walking, swimming

+ Muscular endurance to strengthen the hips, legs, abdomen, chest, and shoulders by performing an average of three sets of ten to twelve repetitions while weight lifting/weight pushing

+ Flexibility exercises by doing stretches and yoga

Exercise has a direct effect on your sexual desire. Furthermore, a low sex drive is frequently caused by stress and fatigue. When you are tired and fatigued, you simply don't have the desire to make love. You think it will take a lot of effort. Exercise, in combination with a healthy, well-balanced, diet can enhance your libido.

Aphrodisiacs

For more than five thousand years, aphrodisiacs have been used to increase sexual powers and a desire for sex. An aphrodisiac is a food, drug, scent, or device that claims to improve libido. They are strongly ingrained in ever culture, yet there is no scientific evidence of what works and what doesn't.

Aphrodisiacs may include such items as foods, herbs, scents, beverages, drugs, or various other potions. Natural aphrodisiacs include vegetables, fruits, nuts, and grains. Antioxidants in certain foods have been credited as a strong aphrodisiac and to have the property to protect against sperm damage. Other compounds, such as sulphur-containing amino acids, L-arginine, L-cysteine, and L-methionine, have been exalted as aphrodisiacs because they maintain blood flow to the sexual organs and increase sperm count.

Here is a list of some foods and spices with possible aphrodisiac properties. Include the following foods in your diet to boost your love life.

Nuts: all kinds

Fruits: bananas, figs, raspberries, strawberries, avocados, grapes, quince, mangos, passion fruit

Vegetables: asparagus, carrots, fennel, celery, chocolate, leeks, beans, radishes, peas

Spices: caraway, cumin, coriander, cardamom seeds, chili, ginger, mustard, cayenne, gingko, cloves, pepper, celery seed, garlic, licorice, nutmeg, saffron

Lose Calories Almost Effortlessly in Small Increments:

Drink Cold Water and Cold Drinks
By drinking cold water and drinks, your body will burn calories to increase the temperature of the drink to your body's temperature. Drinking eight ounces of cold water can burn off approximately ten additional calories as compared to drinking room-temperature water. The potential weight loss is not "a miracle," but, in a year, you could lose as much as five to seven pounds by drinking cold water and making no other changes in your diet. In addition, there might be some other health benefits.

Your body temperature is usually warmer than regular cold drinks. Ice-cold water is below 35° F. This means cold drinks are approximately sixty degrees lower than your body temperature (assuming a 98.6° body temperature)! On average, you have to burn one calorie to raise the temperature of one liter of water 2° F. So, raising the temperature of one liter of cold drink or water to your body temperature requires thirty calories. If you ingest two liters of cold drinks every day, you will burn sixty calories. Of course, a few more calories are needed to absorb and excrete the extra water as urine or sweat. Remember each calorie counts.

Total Calories Burned in One Year by Drinking Two Liters of Ice-Cold Water per Day:

98.6 – 35.6 = 64 calories

(365 days x 64 calories/day = 23,400 calories

23,400 ÷ 9 = 26,000 g of fat = 2.6 kg of fat

2.45 kg fat x 2.2 = 5.7 lbs. of fat

Chew noncaloric gum throughout the day. The act of chewing requires calories, and you can lose ten pounds of body fat in a year.

Keep on Moving

Keep on moving. Keep on moving your limbs. Do self-aware fidgeting as much as you can, whenever you can. You can do this while waiting in line or even waiting online, sitting behind the computer.

Scientists believe that self-aware voluntary movements and activities—such as changing posture, stretching your arms above your head, and getting up from your seat—are responsible for burning many more calories than unconscious fidgeting (290–294). These self-aware and voluntary activities have been termed NEAT (non-exercise activity thermogenesis). It is estimated that NEAT burns from three hundred to eight hundred (289) calories a day. Do more self- aware and natural fidgeting if possible; be more animated!

Breathe better and deeper! When you breathe more naturally and efficiently, it can influence your metabolism greatly and give you an overall sense of well-being. Better oxygenation will burn calories more efficiently and aerobically.

Calories Burned by Different Exercises and Physical Activities

Calories Burned per Hour of Activity	
Sitting, watching TV	100
Standing	140
Making beds	135
Housework	150–250
Strolling	200

Raking leaves	225
Lawn mowing (electric)	250
Lawn-mowing (manual)	300–400
Gardening	150–300
Square dancing	350
Bowling	400
Leisurely swimming	260–750
Brisk swimming	360–500
Doubles tennis	360
Singles tennis	480
Volleyball	300
Softball	280–400
Golf—carrying your own clubs	360
Jogging	600–750
Moderate running	870–1,020
Sprinting	1,130–1,285
Leisurely skating (ice or roller)	400
Fast skating	700
Downhill skiing	500–600
Cross-country skiing	560–1,020
Basketball	300–600
Rowing machine	800

Calories Burned by Common Daily Activities

Calories Burned per Hour of Activity

Lying down or sleeping	50–80
Sitting quietly	60–80
Sitting and writing	90–110
Sitting and card playing	90–120
Gardening	150–325
Light house cleaning	225–250
Walking	200–400

Calories Burned by Common Exercise:

Bicycling	25 cals/mile
Walking	100 cals/mile
Jogging	120 cals/mile
Rowing	125 cals/mile
Skiing	150 cals/mile
Swimming	500 cals/mile
Slow dancing	125 cals/hour
Bowling	150 cals/hour
Gardening	150 cals/hour
Softball	150 cals/hour
Golf	225 cals/hour
Ice-skating	275 cals/hour
Roller-skating	275 cals/hour
Tennis (doubles)	275 cals/hour
Fast dancing	350 cals/hour
Basketball	400 cals/hour
Tennis (singles)	425 cals/hour
Handball	550 cals/hour
Racquetball	550 cals/hour
Rowing machine	750 cals/hour
Jumping rope	850 cals/hour
Stair-climbing	1,050 cals/hour

Target-Heart-Rate Zone

To benefit from the fat-burning effect of aerobic exercises, you need to reach a specified heart rate called the target heart rate zone. This heart rate target has an upper and a lower range. You can calculate this target heart rate as follows.

First, subtract your age from 220 to find out your maximum heart rate. For example, if you are forty years old,

maximum heart rate: 220 minus 40 = 180 beats per minute.

Then, multiply your maximum heart rate by 65 percent to get the lower range of the target zone:

180 minus 65 = 117 beats per minute, lower target zone.

Then, multiply your maximum heart rate by 85 percent to get the higher range of the target zone:

180 x .85 = 153 beats per minute, higher target zone.

So, for a forty-year-old person, target heart rate should reach in the range of 117–153 beats per minute.

When you exercise, your heart rate should be within the optimal target heart rate zone for your age. And in order for you to burn your body fat faster, you should exercise within the lower range. When you exercise at this lower range, you use more fat cells to burn calories.

You can check your heart rate by taking your pulse. Gently place your index and middle finger on the inner part of the wrist. Count how many times your heart beats in ten seconds, and multiply that number by six. You can also obtain a digital heart rate monitor for a nominal price so you can concentrate on your exercises and not taking your pulse.

Chewing and Weight Loss

Chew your food ten to twenty times. You will feel fuller with less food, and it aids digestion. Chew your food longer, as chewing initiates digestion. It is a known fact that overweight people don't chew their food enough, so they produce too little saliva. This means that the stomach is forced to overwork and stretch.

Research has shown that people need to chew—not just drink—in order to feel full and satisfied. In addition, you can burn some extra calories by chewing solid food. Raw food, primarily vegetables and fruits, are fashionable and healthy for you. Munching down on fresh vegetables like carrots, celery, green peppers, cucumbers, and broccoli can provide you with a satisfying and satiating crunch.

Chapter Seven

Let's Start

Hopefully you have read all the chapters and have decided to make the L.O.V.E. diet part of your life. Now you are ready to start the program. It is a good idea to incorporate all the ideas and recommendations into your lifestyle.

First, we will go over a short review of the nutrition points. As mentioned before, it is extremely important to know something about the food that you ingest. This will require you to learn and know some basic nutrition (refer to chapter 2). You also need to read food labels.

Let's Review

You have come up with ways to improve your diet and reduce overall caloric intake, and will do the following:

pick foods from the low-Glycemic Index list

try to eat smaller portions, but eat more frequently and do not skip any meals, especially breakfast

Your daily intake will be:

+ 55 percent carbohydrates

+ 30 percent oils/fats

+ 15 percent proteins

You have decided to eliminate or at least reduce the amount of the bad oils/fats in your diet and have picked several good cooking oils and fats. You've also selected several varieties of nuts to add to your diet.

You have decided to go to your supermarket or your local farmer's market and select large amounts of vegetables, fruits, and herbs. Shop more often to ensure getting freshest food. You will try some exotic fruits and vegetables, and always attempt to mix different types of these foods, as no single vegetable, fruit, herb, or nut will be nutritious enough. In fact, no single food will deliver all the nutrients your body requires.

You have decided to eat more salads—salads full of color, not just lettuce alone. You will use olive oil and vinegar/lemon juice.

You will try to avoid factory-made dressings.

You will drink eight to ten glasses of water per day.

You have picked several forms of activities to do throughout the day.

Short Course in Good Nutrition

Remember, you gain weight if and only if you take in too many calories. Don't dramatically restrict your intake of carbohydrates, protein, or fat. Carbohydrates do not make you fat (make carbohydrates 55 percent of your diet). Proteins do not make you fat (15 percent of your dietary intake should be proteins). Fats do not make you fat (30 percent of your daily diet should be fats/oils).

Include some carbohydrates, protein, and fat in every meal. Eat the right food, and don't starve.

Remember: what you eat and drink impacts how you look, feel, and perform. Nourish your body rather than fill it with empty, bad calories.

Eliminate bad calories that contain no nutritional value.

Eliminate bad drinks like soda, filtered fruit juices, and energy drinks. Drink water instead.

Eat smaller portions, and eat more frequently (grazing).

Avoid eating fast food, but if you have to, order foods with good nutritional value. Eliminate deep-fried foods.

Limit your intake of high- and medium-Glycemic Index foods, such as potatoes and pastas.

Increase intake of low-Glycemic Index foods, such as fruits, vegetables, herbs, and whole-wheat breads.

Eat fewer calories per day.

Things You Should Do More Often to Lose More Weight

+ Eat fewer calories per day.
+ Eat more vegetables, fruits, complex carbohydrates, and whole grains.
+ Eat more of the low-Glycemic Index foods.
+ Eat better quality oils but fewer fats.
+ Eat more foods that are high in vitamins A, C, E, B, and folic acid.
+ Drink more water.
+ Limit coffee and soft drinks.
+ Eliminate sugar, refined foods, preserved foods, and fat-laden snack foods.
+ Always think positively.
+ Eliminate all negative thoughts, and change your attitude for the better.
+ Remember the concept of "mind over body."
+ Don't forget that you are a composite of mind, body, and soul.

A Successful Weight-Loss and Weight-Management Program

Successful weight-loss and weight-management programs depend on reasonable goals and expectations. If you set reasonable goals for yourself, you'll be more likely to meet them and have a better chance of keeping off the weight lost. Even a modest weight loss of 5 to 10 percent can help improve your health (295–297).

It is also a good practice to lose your extra weight gradually. Generally, you should avoid losing more than two pounds per week. If, for any health-related reason, a more rapid weight loss is recommended for you, you should be under the direct supervision of a physician. This is essential for your safety.

Major factors in a successful weight-loss program are realistic goals, behavioral modification, regular physical activity, calorie reduction, healthful eating, and avoidance of hunger. Successful weight loss and weight management should address all of these factors.

Gradual Weight Loss Is Preferred

Most physicians and health professionals advocate a gradual weight-loss program as the safest and most successful approach. Gradual weight loss encourages loss of body fat, not just water weight. A reasonable weight-loss program allows you to lose approximately one pound of weight per week. As a rule, the majority of people who are moderately active will require approximately fifteen calories per pound to maintain their weight. For example, a two-hundred-pound person needs to take in three thousand calories to maintain his or her weight. To shed one pound of extra weight, a person must burn thirty-five hundred calories more than taken in. For example, reducing calories by a combination of eating fewer calories and increasing daily activity to burn off additional calories should result in a weight loss of one pound per week.

Okay. Now, you need to find out your ideal weight and evaluate your goals. The first and most important question is: are you overweight, obese, or morbidly obese? This will require you to calculate your ideal weight.

So, Are You Obese or Overweight?

According to the latest scientific definition, you are considered obese if your body weight is 20 percent more than the ideal weight for a person of your height. You are considered overweight if you are 10 percent above the scientifically defined ideal weight (276). According to these definitions, a muscular person can also be characterized as overweight while having a very low percentage of body fat. Therefore, body weight alone is not an accurate gauge of obesity.

How to Determine Your Optimal Weight

The first step is to figure out your body mass index (BMI), which is a reliable way to estimate your body fat and the health risks associated with being overweight or obese. BMI is reliable for most people between the ages of eighteen and seventy years. Of course, in certain groups of people, such as pregnant or breast-feeding women and chronically ill individuals, it is not reliable.

BMI is a measure of body weight that factors in a person's height when determining levels. There are five main levels of BMI.

- BMI of 19 or less is considered underweight

- BMI of 20–25 is the ideal weight

- BMI of 26–30 is overweight

- BMI of 31–40 is obese

- BMI of 41 and higher is morbidly obese

In general, the higher your BMI, the higher your health risk. In addition to BMI, there is a very simple factor that can easily be measured—the waistline. The risk of a high BMI increases if your waist size is greater than forty inches (for a man) or thirty-five inches (for a woman). Refer to the BMI chart (on page) and use it to determine your current BMI, and your optimal weight and its corresponding optimal BMI, which should be lower than 26. Then, measure your waist. Now, look at the chart on page 00 to determine your health risk relative to normal weight.

Risk of Disease Associated with BMI and Waist Size			
BMI	Weight type	Waist less than or equal to 40 in. (men) or 35 in. (women)	Waist greater than 40 in. (men) or 35 in. (women)
18.5 or less	Underweight	—	—
18.5–24.9	Normal	—	—
25.0–29.9	Overweight	Increased	High
30.0–34.9	Obese	High	Very High
35.0–39.9	Obese	Very High	Very High
40 or greater	Extremely Obese	Extremely High	Extremely High

- Determine your weight.

- Determine your height.

- Determine your BMI (use the chart on page 00).

- Determine your waistline.

+ Determine your risk of disease.

Now you can also calculate your ideal weight according to the following formula (see page 00). Set a clear goal for the number of pounds you want to lose based on this calculation or from the above chart. Make sure that you set realistic goals for your weight-loss program and, most important, that your anticipated rate of weight loss is reasonable.

Now, based on your ideal weight, calculate your caloric requirement per day, meaning your basal metabolic rate. It is important to know this number, so you can curb your diet to this level.

Obesity and Health

Obesity is a serious disease with serious health risks. According to the US surgeon general, an estimated three hundred thousand deaths per year may be attributable to obesity (298– 300). The risk of death rises with increasing weight. Even being moderately overweight (ten to twenty pounds in a average person) increases the risk of death, particularly among adults aged thirty to sixty-five.

Overweight and obesity are strongly linked with an increased risk for some types of cancer, including breast, colon, gallbladder, and prostate cancers. For example, women double their risk of postmenopausal breast cancer if they gain more than twenty pounds between the ages of eighteen to midlife compared to women whose weight remains stable (301, 302).

Weight Loss and Health

Individuals with a BMI greater than 30 (obese) have a greater than 70 percent increased risk of premature death from all causes. The degree of increased risk factor depends on how obese the individual is. A modest weight loss of 5 percent to 15 percent of total body weight in an individual with a BMI greater than 30 reduces the risk factors for some diseases, particularly heart disease.

First, you need to approximate your ideal weight using the following simple formula.

Ideal Weight Range for Women

1. Give yourself one hundred pounds for five feet of height.

2. Add five pounds for each additional inch.

3. Adjust the value in part 2 for different frame sizes (based on your height and/or clothing size):

+ Petite: add 3 percent.

+ Small: add 5 percent.

+ Medium: add 7 percent.

+ Large: add 9 percent.

Ideal Weight Range for Men

1. Start with 110 pounds for five feet of height.

2. Add six pounds for each additional inch.

3. Adjust the value in part (2) for different frame sizes:

+ Petite: add 4 percent.

+ Small: add 6 percent.

+ Medium: add 8 percent.

+ Large: add 10 percent.

Calculating Your BMR

There are two ways you can calculate your BMR (see page 00)

1. The Harris Benedict formula.

2. An alternative and simple way to calculate your BMR.

How to Start the L.O.V.E. Diet Program

You should start with thinking positively. Accept yourself as who you are, but recognize you have huge potential and need to achieve that potential.

Take control of your life and your life situation. This may not be easy, but it is achievable. Always think positively, and eliminate all negative thoughts. Change your attitude for the better. Remember the concept of mind over body, but don't forget that you are a composite of mind, body, and soul. All these elements need to be given appropriate attention, so go on and meditate and get in touch with you. Learn to relax. Remember, you don't need any negative energy, because it will also affect your self-esteem. Be good to yourself. Let yourself enjoy life. Try to do things that make you happy. Dress up for you. Keep on reminding yourself that you will be able to attain a better physical appearance. Eat natural foods and exercise. And don't forget to tell yourself, "I love you." Always set realistic and achievable goals, and as soon as you reach them, reward yourself and set future goals.

The L.O.V.E. Diet

The L.O.V.E. diet requires a high intake of fruits, vegetables, whole grains, beans, nuts, pasta, rice, and seeds. Olive oil consumption, with other dairy products in moderate amounts in the form of cheese and yogurt, makes up the remainder of this diet. Of course, a small amount of lean animal proteins are included. This diet has a moderate fat content—the good fat.

You should include no more than 25 percent to 30 percent of your daily caloric intake from fat. You should avoid saturated fats; the majority of fat should be from the good fats. Substitute refined carbohydrates with complex carbohydrates to decrease the calories consumed. Consume more foods with high fiber intake which have not been refined. And increase your physical activity. You should try to lower your LDL cholesterol and increase your HDL cholesterol by eliminating bad fats and incorporating the good fats found in avocados, nuts, fish, and other healthy foods.

This diet takes advantage of the soybean, which, in the last five years or so, has been given a lot of positive press. Soy is a protein-packed food that, depending on what you want, can replace meat or dairy. By substituting soy for some of your animal-based meals, you can reduce your risk for heart disease. Plant-derived proteins, like those found in soy, lower LDL cholesterol and raise HDL cholesterol. This prevents hardening of the arteries (atherosclerosis) and heart disease, thus reducing the risk of stroke and heart attack. Additionally, plant-based protein diets enhance calcium retention in the body and results in less excretion of calcium in the urine.

This reduces the risk of osteoporosis and development of kidney stones and kidney dysfunction (1–5, 303–309). Kidney disease is far less common in people who eat a plant-based diet than it is in people who eat an animal-based diet (310–318), so you should attempt to replace animal protein with vegetable protein in addition to replacing saturated fat with unsaturated fat, which can be found in plant/seed-derived oils like olive and canola oils.

The benefits of a low-fat diet include a reduced chance of heart disease and certain cancers, increased energy and brain productivity, and healthy, long-term weight maintenance.

Increase your intake of foods high in fiber. This will fill you up without making you gain weight. A high-fiber diet will stabilize your blood sugar, lower cancer risk, and control your appetite. A large variety of healthy and delicious foods are high in fiber.

The typical American diet is loaded with sodium. Low sodium diets, such as the DASH diet, limit sodium intake to twenty-four milligrams per day. Nevertheless, reducing sodium does not in any way mean food is bland or tasteless! In this diet, fresh herbs, spices, and other healthy foods are encouraged to add zest to foods while eliminating the salt. It has been proven that a low-salt diet, in combination with the DASH diet, controls blood pressure, thereby reducing the need to take medications for high blood pressure. In addition, heart function can be improved, and fluid retention is reduced.

Things You Need to Start the Diet of L.O.V.E Program

So, now you want to start this holistic diet to attain a better health status and healthier weight which is ideal for you. In order to achieve your goal, you need to the following:

My Diet of L.O.V.E. Contract

The Diet of L.O.V.E. Weight-Loss Contract

I, _____, promise to commit myself to the L.O.V.E. diet and follow its teachings through its ten commandments. I do this because I love and respect myself.

I, _____, am ready to take control of my life and my health by starting a realistic weight-loss program that will include a reduced-calorie diet and increased physical activity.

I, _____, realize that the weight-loss/weight-control program is a significant issue in improving my fitness and ultimately my health. I also realize that there are serious health risks that are associated with being overweight. Therefore, I'm very serious and completely enthusiastic to change my lifestyle so that I can improve my health and well-being.

I, _____, am fully committed to my success and can't wait to get started! To achieve this, I am signing this contract, which is a behavioral change contract that will set specific and attainable goals for me.

I, _____, will set these goals, and I will revise them whenever I reach either the set goals or every six months, whichever comes first.

I, _____, am well aware of the fact that I may get frustrated easily with my diet and weight-loss program, but I will not allow this frustration to defeat my efforts.

_____   _____
(Signature)   (Date)

My Diet of L.O.V.E. Worksheet

+ Measure your height and your weight.

+ Calculate the ideal weight for your gender, frame, and height.

+ Look up your current BMI in the chart.

+ Look up your ideal BMI in the chart.

+ Look up your ideal weight for your height and frame.

+ Subtract your current weight from your ideal weight.

+ This gives you the total extra weight that you need to lose.

+ Divide the extra weight by 1 (lower range of number of weeks needed to lose your extra weight without severe stress).

+ Divide the extra weight by 2 (upper range of number of weeks needed to lose your extra weight without severe stress).

+ Take the value of your extra weight and multiply it by 3,500 calories per pound of fat.

+ Divide the value of total calories by the lower range of number of weeks.

+ Then divide it by 7.

+ Divide the value of total calories by upper range of number of weeks.

+ Now divide it by 7.

Personalized Worksheet

A) My current weight (pounds)_____

B) My height (inches)_____

C) My current BMI_____

D) My desired BMI_____

E) My target weight for my desired BMI_____

F) Calculate your extra weight:

Current weight (A)_____ – Target weight (E)_____ = Extra weight (F)

G) Calculate the maximum number of weeks needed to lose your extra weight: Extra weight ÷ 1

H) Calculate the minimum number of weeks needed to lose your extra weight: Extra weight ÷ 2

I) To calculate the total number of calories in that extra weight, take the value for your extra weight (F) and multiply it by 3,500 (number of calories per pound of fat):

Extra weight (F)_____x 3,500 = total number of calories

J) To calculate the minimum number of calories needed to burn per week, divide the value of total number of calories (I) by maximum number of weeks (G):

Total number of calories (I) _____÷ maximum number of weeks (G)

K) To calculate the maximum number of calories needed to burn per week, divide the value of total number of calories (I) by minimum number of weeks (H):

Total number of calories (I)_____÷ minimum number of weeks (H)

L) To calculate the minimum number of calories to burn per day to lose extra weight, divide the value of minimum number of calories per week (J) by 7:

Minimum total number of calories per week (J)_____÷ 7

M) To calculate maximum number of calories to burn per day to lose extra weight, divide the value of maximum total number of calories per week (K) by 7:

Maximum total number of calories per week (K)_____÷ 7

My Diet of L.O.V.E Plan in Summary

Therefore, you will need to lose a range of (L)_____to
(M)_____number of calories per day to lose your extra weight
(F)_____in a range of (H)_____to (G)_____weeks,
without stressing your body and jeopardizing your health.

Example:

Take a forty-year-old man who weighs 190 lbs. and is 5 feet
8 inches tall. Current weight = 190 lbs

Height = 5 foot 8 inches = 68 inches

Current BMI (see chart) = 29 (obese dangerous weight)
Desired BMI = 25

Target weight for the desired BMI = 164 lbs.

Current weight (190) − Target weight (164) = 26 lbs. of
extra weight

190 − 164 = 26 lbs. extra weight

Value of (A) = 26

Lower range of number of weeks needed to lose your extra
weight: Extra weight (26 lbs.)

÷ 1 = 26 weeks required to lose the weight at 1 pound per
week

Value of (B) = 26

Upper range of number of weeks needed to lose your extra
weight: Extra weight (26 lbs)

÷ 2 = 13 weeks required to lose the weight at 2 pounds per week

Value of (C) = 13

Take the value for your extra weight (A) and multiply it by 3,500 calories per pound of fat.

26 x 3, 500 = 91,000

Value of (D) = 91,000: this is the number of total calories to be burned in a period of 13 to 26 weeks to lose the extra 26 pounds!

Divide the value of (D) by (B)

91,000 ÷ 26 = 3,500 calories

Value of (E) = 3,500: this is the number of calories to burn per week in a course of 26 weeks

Divide the value of (D) by 13

91,000 ÷ 13 = 7,000 calories

Value of (F) = 7,000: this is the number of calories to burn per week in a course of 13 weeks

Divide the value of (E) by 7

3,500 ÷ 7 = 500

Value of (G) = 500: this is the number of calories he has to lose per day to lose 26 pounds of extra weight in 26 weeks!

Divide the value of (F) by 7

7,000 ÷ 7 = 1,000

Value of (H) = 1,000: this is the number of calories he has to lose per day to lose 26 pounds of extra weight in 13 weeks!

You need to lose a range of (G) to (H) calories per day to love your weight in a range of (B) to (C) weeks, without stressing your body and jeopardizing your health.

My Diet of L.O.V.E. Weight-Loss Program
Based on My Desired Weight

I currently weigh (A) _____, and based on my current weight and height (B) _____, my calculated BMI is (C) _____. This puts me in the category of _____ Obese, _____ Overweight, _____ Slightly overweight person.

Therefore, my optimal weight based on an optimal BMI of 25 or lower is (D) _____. Based on my optimal weight, I am (F) _____ pounds heavier than my optimal weight of (E) _____.

In order to lose my extra weight (F) _____, I have to lose a total of (I)_____ calories in a period of at least (G) _____ weeks to a maximum of (H) _____ weeks to avoid stressing my health and body.

This calculates to a minimum of (L) _____ calories per day to a maximum of (M)_____ calories per day.

My pledge and promise to myself is as follows

I, _____, will give my L.O.V.E. diet program a top priority and will try to incorporate it into my life. I recognize that any successful weight-loss program requires me to be committed to changing my lifestyle.

I, _____, realize the following:

I need to lose _____ lbs. of weight. This will take time and effort.

I realize and agree to achieve my goal of _____ pounds weight loss by adopting the following:

Physical Activity:

Because physical activity is an important part of weight management and overall health,

+ I will engage in physical activity _____ times per week for _____ minutes.
+ I will also increase my activities as follows:

Dance more
Sing more often
Walk more
Gardening more often

Shop /window shopping more often
Belly dance more
Chew my meald thoroughly and longer

Eat

+ I will limit my intake to _____ calories per day.

+ I will start eating low Glycemic Index foods, such as _____.

+ I will avoid eating high and medium glycemic foods, such as _____.

+ I will start using good oils and eat more nuts every day, such as _____.

Drink

+ I will limit my drinks to no more than one per day, if any.

+ I will start drinking about eight to ten glasses of pure water per day.

+ I will avoid drinking high sugar drinks and fast food.

Take a multivitamin

+ I will take one multivitamin pill a day.

Sleep

I will sleep a minimum of _____ hours per night. I will adjust my sleep time as needed to get a restful sleep.

Relax

I will do the following to relax my mind and body:

+ Take a bubble bath.

+ Listen to music.

+ Sing.

- Get a massage.
- Take advantage of aromatherapy.
- Get a facial.

Get more antioxidants into my diet

- I will increase my antioxidant intake by eating more of (choose from the table 00 on page 00)

Rewards

I will reward myself as follows:

- increase my antioxidant intake by eating more of (choose from the table on page 00)

- I will receive _____ as a reward every time I reach a new weight target _____ 3 lbs. _____ 5 lbs. _____ 10 lbs. _____ lbs., or whenever I am successful in maintaining my new weight target for 4 weeks.

My short-term goal is _____

_____.

My long-term goal is _____

_____.

Signature _____

Date _____

Rate Your Own Plate

Get into the habit of rating your own plate and, thereby, attempt different ways that you can improve your plate by making healthier food choices.

Which foods would you choose?

Entrée _____ Side Dish ___ Side Dish ___ Beverage ____ Dessert _____

Calories ____ Calories ____ Calories ____ Calories ____ Calories ____

What is the total amount of nutrients in your meal?
Calories?
Total fat?
Antioxidants?

An Example of a Healthy Diet

Breakfast

1 cup of cut fruit (strawberries, melons, pineapple, grapes, etc.) or a whole fruit
1/2 cup low-fat cottage cheese or 1/2 cup of yogurt
1 slice of whole-grain, high-fiber, or multigrain toast

Mid-morning Snack

1 medium fruit (not a fruit juice), like banana, apple, or orange
Or 1–2 ounces (a handful) of any nut

Lunch

A big bowl of salad, consisting of multi-colored varieties of vegetables and fruits with different, for example, dark green lettuce; broccoli; cauliflower;

tomatoes; red, yellow, or green peppers; carrots, with two teaspoons of walnut oil
2 ounces organic beef patty served on a whole-grain roll

Mid-afternoon Snack

Some cut vegetables, like carrot sticks and celery, plus 1 ounce of nuts or seeds

Dinner

Small portion of starch (1/2 cup of whole-wheat spaghetti or high-fiber toast)
Or 2 ounces of plant-based protein (soy, tofu) or animal-based protein (meat, chicken, or fish)
2 cups of cooked green vegetables, such as asparagus, spinach, or broccoli or regular salad drizzled with a dressing of 5 to 6 teaspoons of lemon juice and 2 teaspoons of olive oil, grapeseed oil, or flaxseed oil.

Evening Snack

1 1/2 ounce of cheese and 1 medium fruit

Make sure you drink plenty of water (eight glasses). Feel free to add some lemon juice or low-calorie artificial flavors if you like.

Chapter Eight

Let's Stop the Aging Process Now!

The Aging Process—Aging Is Inevitable!

The subject of aging and the fountain of youth dates back to biblical times. Physicians and scientists have long sought to understand and describe the mechanisms of the aging process. The aging process begins in utero, as early as the moment of conception. This process is an inevitable course, and no one alive is immune to it. You and your body, as a living organism, go through the aging process every minute of your life. In general, your body reaches its peak efficiency about age thirty and then begins to decline afterward. However, some people "age" at a slower rate and endure the aging process better. The good news is that even though this process of aging is unavoidable, you can slow its progression drastically. You can live a healthier lifestyle and slow the aging process. You'll be able to have a high-quality and long life by reducing aging's negative aspects and promoting its positive aspects.

As your body ages, it goes through many changes. All your organs are affected, and each one is impacted differently. Since each organ system has its own function, each reacts to the aging process based on its physiological functions. Your muscle mass decreases, and your bones become brittle. In addition, your immune system weakens, and you cannot fight disease and injury as well as when younger. Of course, other functions, such as hearing, eyesight, and reflexes, may also be affected.

How and Why Do You Age?

Your tissues and organs are made up of numerous kinds of cells that function harmoniously. There are nearly a trillion—a million million—cells in your body. These cells are the smallest building blocks of your body. They carry the vital processes needed to sustain life and maintain your health. When scientists unravel the mechanisms of how and why cells age, how they lose their ability to function and reproduce and then ultimately die, it may help us understand and cure all the age-related diseases and conditions.

To understand the aging process and its mechanisms, scientists have been looking deep into our cells, seeking clues to these complex questions. There are several scientific theories postulated to explain this complex and unavoidable process. Since the completion of the Human Genome Project has unraveled the makeup of the genetic, molecular, and other biological processes of the human body and cells, we have been able to hone in on some major mechanisms. One of the major theories of aging is the free radical theory. But before explaining this important theory we need to discuss two very important terms: oxidation and free radicals.

What Is Oxidation?

Oxidation is a reaction of any substance or compound with the molecules of oxygen. This natural process occurs around us and in our bodies all the time. Rusting is a prime example of oxidation. Many biological and biochemical reactions in our bodies consist of a reaction called oxidation-reduction. Via this reaction, one substance or molecule becomes "oxidized," while another one becomes "reduced." Oxidation is part of every living organism, and there is no way to avoid it. The oxidative reaction produces harmful chemicals known as free radicals, which subsequently damage and weaken the important content of your cells. Through oxidation, the cells and organs in your body can be made weak, which can lead to diseases like cancer and heart disease as well as aging.

What Are Free Radicals?

Free radicals are highly unstable molecules that are generated mainly during the process of oxidation; the very process that produces the energy necessary to stay alive. They also come from outside sources, such as environmental pollution, smoking, and various synthetic chemicals that are added to our water and food.

Free radicals are chemically unstable because they lack one electron. In order to stabilize themselves, they attack any other substance within their reach and grab an electron from them. This, of course, creates a new free radical, which proceeds to repeat the process, producing a domino effect. When this reaction is uncontrolled, it can generate millions of free radicals within seconds.

Free radicals are oxygen molecules that are produced either naturally as by-products of metabolism or purposefully to destroy and kill harmful microbes and bacteria. There are many types of free radicals. Some are environmental, and some are ingested with foods. Yet another group is formed within the body.

Free radicals are highly reactive and unstable molecules, and, therefore, they are very harmful if not kept under control. They can cause disease by damaging cells in your body. They are highly toxic, because they damage the information center cells in your body—the DNA of your cells—and oxidize vital molecules and proteins in your body.

Free radicals play a major role in many diseases, from Alzheimer's to heart disease to retinal disease. In the body, this oxidative damage by free radicals is a major contributor to the development of cancer. Recent research indicates that free radical damage may be the basis for the aging process as well (319–325).

These free radicals damage key enzymes, cell membranes and even the DNA—the genetic material. According to some estimates, free radicals can be linked to over sixty diseases, including diabetes, heart disease, Alzheimer's disease, cancers, and arthritis. They can cause severe reduction in cell function and even the death of a cell.

Scientists have been investigating how antioxidants and foods rich in antioxidants can reduce and neutralize the harmful effects of oxidative damage caused by the free radicals and, thereby, slow the aging process (319–224)

The Free Radical Theory of Aging

Free radical theory of aging—also known as damage theory—is based on the scientific fact there is an accumulation of damages inside the cells of your body as a process of aging. These damages are secondary to the effects of free radicals generated in your body and cells over time as part of the oxidation processes (see page 00). Free radicals and the damage they cause to your cells are believed to be the underlying causes of aging and aging-related diseases, like many types of cancer and Alzheimer's disease. Therefore, the theory holds that the aging process may be (most likely is) the result of the accumulation of structural damage to our cells from continuously formed free radicals in our bodies and cells (319–326).

Aging and Nutrition

It is well known that as you age, the nutritional requirement of your body changes—sometimes drastically. For example, when you are younger, your digestive system and metabolism are more robust, and you can digest and utilize macronutrients and micronutrients more efficiently. As you age, your metabolism, digestive, and absorption processes do not function optimally. Some foods, however, hold solutions to slowing the aging of our bodies and maintaining a healthy longer life span.

Antioxidants

These potent agents can reduce the cumulative damages from free radicals, thereby reducing the rate of many leading diseases, such as cancer.

Many substances, such as phytochemicals, as well as many vitamins found in all vegetables and fruit act as antioxidants. Vitamin C, vitamin E, and beta-carotene (which changes to vitamin A in the body) are all antioxidants. It is best to choose foods high in these vitamins rather than take vitamin supplements.

Experts say that it may not be the vitamins that specifically help protect against cancer. The health benefits may be due to the natural combination of these vitamins with other important nutrients, such as phytochemicals and fibers found in these foods.

Phytochemicals are natural plant compounds that can reduce the risk of cancer. There is some evidence that different phytochemicals may help prevent the formation of hazardous carcinogens, substances that cause or promote cancer. In addition, it is believed they may also block the action of carcinogens on their target organs and ultimately suppress cancer development (326). All vegetables and fruit contain phytochemicals. As a rule, darker green, red, and orange vegetables and fruit are particularly rich in phytochemicals.

Since vegetables and fruit play a key role in a healthy diet, add the following colourful vegetables and fruits to your diet: broccoli, spinach, sweet potatoes, squash, red and yellow peppers, cantaloupe, citrus fruits, all types of berries, and tomatoes. But always wash your vegetables and fruits well with running water. Scrub the skin well if it is edible.

All About Antioxidants

Everyone needs antioxidants to help prevent damage to their body caused by free radicals. These unstable molecules, through a self-perpetuating chain reaction, cause millions of new free radicals that damage proteins, cells, tissues, and organs. They cause aging, degenerative changes, inflammation, and disease. They cut short your life span.

Antioxidants prevent damage by protecting the proteins, cells, tissues, and organs that are targeted by free radicals. Antioxidants have been scientifically proven to (319–326):

+ Prevent aging

+ Prevent heart disease

+ Prevent a variety of cancers

+ Prevent blindness

+ Boost the immune system

Antioxidants Occur Naturally in Food Sources

Even though fruits and vegetables are loaded with antioxidants, not all of them are equal in power and strength. USDA scientists have developed a method to measure the ability of antioxidants in any substance, including certain foods and your blood, to neutralize and subdue free radicals. This method is called the Oxygen Radical Absorbance Capacity (ORAC), which is a measurement of the substance to neutralize and subdue oxygen free radicals.

ORAC: Oxygen Radical Absorbance Capacity

USDA scientists have demonstrated that increasing your intake of fruits and vegetables with high ORAC factors is an effective way to fight free radicals and, thereby, slowing the aging process and its complications. It is interesting that researchers have found that vitamins C and E can, in the presence of transition metals such as copper or iron ions, become oxidizing agents themselves! This effect was not seen when the whole fruit or vegetable extract was pitted against copper ions. It was also demonstrated that the antioxidant power in fruits and vegetables come from other substances in addition to their vitamin content.

ORAC values are higher in dark colored fruits and vegetables than in lighter colored ones, suggesting that color may contain essential beneficial compounds.

Another study has shown that if you double your intake of fruits and vegetables from five servings to ten servings, your ORAC can double (1,600 units vs. 3,400).

ORAC Is a Unique Method

There are several methods that measure the total antioxidant capacity of any biological sample. But the ORAC method is unique. ORAC integrates the measurements of the degree and the time that it takes an antioxidant to inhibit the action of an oxidizing agent into one value. This provides an accurate and reproducible measurement for different types of antioxidants having different strengths.

Which Antioxidants Are Needed?

Getting a variety of antioxidants is important, because each antioxidant targets certain types of damaging free radicals. Getting a variety will help cover all of your health bases.

A

Alpha-lipoic Acid

Alpha-lipoic acid (ALA)—also known as lipoic acid or thioctic acid—is a vitamin-like antioxidant, sometimes referred to as the "universal antioxidant," because it is soluble in both fat and water. ALA is manufactured in the body and found in animal and plant sources. It is found in spinach, liver, and brewer's yeast. Canola oil, ground flaxseed, and walnuts are rich sources of ALA.

ALA is a highly potent antioxidant that may help protect against atherosclerosis and may help slow the progression of diabetic neuropathy and HIV. ALA provides a double benefit by regenerating and recycling other important antioxidants, such as vitamin C, vitamin E, coenzyme Q10, and glutathione.

C

Carotenoids

Carotenoids are a class of natural, fat-soluble pigments found principally in plants and algae. Carotenoids are responsible for many of the red, orange, and yellow hues of vegetables and fruits. Some familiar examples of carotenoid coloration are the oranges of carrots and citrus fruits, the reds of peppers and tomatoes, and the pinks of salmon. Of the more than seven hundred naturally occurring carotenoids identified thus far, as many as fifty may be absorbed and metabolized by the human body. To date, only fourteen carotenoids have been identified in human serum. Beta-carotene, the principal carotenoid in carrots, is a familiar carotene, while lutein is the major yellow pigment of vegetables and fruit. In human beings, carotenoids can serve several important functions. The most widely studied and well-understood nutritional role for carotenoids is their pro-vitamin activity.

Carotenoids are absorbed from the intestine with the aid of dietary fat. Due to their fat-solubility character, carotenoids are associated with fatty portions of human tissues, cells, and membranes. In general, 80 percent of carotenoids are distributed in body fat, with smaller amounts found in the liver, muscle, adrenal glands, and reproductive organs. Approximately 1 percent circulates in the serum in HDL and LDL cholesterols. The major serum carotenoids are beta-carotene, alpha-carotene, lutein, zeaxanthin, and lycopene.

Catechins (see Flavanoids)
Coenzyme Q10 (CoQ10)

Coenzyme Q10 (CoQ10) is a member of the ubiquinone family. CoQ10 is considered a nonessential nutrient, as our bodies can synthesize it. It is found in small amounts in a wide variety of foods and is synthesized in all tissues. This fat-soluble antioxidant also takes part in energy production in the body's cells. The body produces CoQ10, but production decreases with age. CoQ10 may be beneficial for heart disease, such as reducing the risk of congestive heart failure and/or heart attack.

CoQ10 also acts as an antioxidant, protecting us from free radical damage. Its antioxidant effects are similar to those of vitamin E. Some studies also suggest that CoQ10 may boost the immune system.

E

Ellagic Acid (see Flavonoids)
Epicatechins (see Flavonoids)

F

Flavonoids

More than four thousand flavonoids have been identified in plants, and many are antioxidants. Flavonoids are a group of chemical compounds naturally found in certain fruits, vegetables, teas, wines, nuts, and seeds. They not only have antioxidant properties but also have anti-inflammatory properties. Flavonoids have been shown to prevent or slow the development of some cancers. Flavonoids are usually subdivided into five subgroups:

1. Flavonols: Quercetin, Kaempferol, Myricetin, and Isorhamnetin

Quercetin has a potent antioxidant activity that may play a role in protection against cancer. It may have beneficial effects on immune function, allergies, stomach health, and diabetic complications, such as cataracts and neuropathy. It has also been shown to have anti- inflammatory properties.

2. Flavones: Luteolin, Apigenin
3. Flavanones: Hesperidin, Naringenin, Eriodictyol

Hesperidin is a member of the flavonoid family and has been shown to have antioxidant activity. It may be beneficial for circulatory and heart health.

4. Flavan-3-ols: Catechin, Gallocatechin, Epicatechin, Epigallocatechin, Theaflavin, Thearubigins

Catechins and epicatechins are strong antioxidants that may protect against cancer and atherosclerosis and may also have anti-inflammatory benefits. These compounds improve blood flow and, thus, are good for cardiac health. Cocoa, particularly dark chocolate, is loaded with the flavonoid epicatechin and has been found to have nearly twice the antioxidants of red wine and up to three times those found in green tea. Green tea contains the most potent catechin, epigallocatechin.

5. Anthocyanidins: Cyanidin, Delphinidin, Malvidin, Pelargonidin, Peonidin, Petunidin

Ellagic Acid

Ellagic acid is a naturally occurring phytochemical found in a variety of plant species. Ellagic acid is a phenolic compound, which acts as a powerful antioxidant. In addition, this compound prevents the binding of carcinogens to DNA and reduces the incidence of cancer in cultured human cells exposed to carcinogens. Ellagic acid is widely found in plants such as raspberries, strawberries, blackberries, cranberries, walnuts, and pecans, but the greatest amounts have been observed in raspberries. While the leaves of these plants contain the highest concentrations of ellagic acid, the compound is also found in their fruits and nuts.

Even though ellagic acid is the bioactive agent that offers protection, the phytochemical is generally ingested in the form of another biochemical called ellagitannins. Plants produce ellagic acid and glucose that combine to form ellagitannins, which are water-soluble compounds that are easier for humans to absorb in their diets. Therefore, small amounts of ellagitannins derived from natural sources may be more effective in the human diet than large doses of purified ellagic acid.

G

Grapeseed Extract

Grapeseed is derived from the seeds and skins of red grapes. Grapeseed extract contains compounds called oligomeric proanthocyanidins (OPC) and proanthocyanidins (PCO), which are powerful antioxidants. In addition to their antioxidant properties, PCO in grapeseed extract have also been shown to improve blood circulation and help to strengthen blood vessels. This is important for individuals with conditions such as varicose veins, leg cramps, arm or leg numbness, and even diabetes. Grapeseed extract may be helpful for those with vascular (vessel) disorders, who may benefit from an increase in blood flow. Grapeseed extract may also be beneficial in reducing inflammation.

These chemicals are potent antioxidants that may protect against heart disease and cancer. They also may have an anti-inflammatory effect.

Oligomeric Proanthocyanidins (OPC) and Proanthocyanidins Oligomers (PCO) are a group of closely related compounds with powerful antioxidant activity, which can reduce the damage done by free radicals, repair connective tissue, and promote enzyme activity. OPC can also help moderate allergic and inflammatory responses by reducing histamine production. Foods that contain this group of chemicals are grapeseed oil, red wine, cranberries, blueberries, bilberries, tea (green and black), black currants, onions, legumes, and parsley.

L

Lutein

Lutein is an antioxidant of the carotenoid family. Lutein can be found in found in yellow and dark green leafy vegetables, such as spinach, collards, kale and broccoli, various fruits, and corn. Egg yolks are also sources of lutein.

Lutein and zeaxanthin are two antioxidant nutrients found highly concentrated in the macula. They give the macula its characteristic yellow appearance. Lutein is strongly associated with a reduced risk of cataracts and macular degeneration.

Lycopene

Lycopene is a bright red carotenoid pigment found in all the red fruits, including tomatoes, and is the most common carotenoid in the human body. Lycopene is not produced in the body, so you can only obtain its benefits by eating foods rich in lycopene. The highest natural concentrations of lycopene are found not in tomatoes but in watermelon. Food processing increases the potency of lycopene, a powerful antioxidant. Cooking tomatoes increases the bioavailability of lycopene and promotes isomerization to antioxidant forms of the chemical. Ongoing research suggests that lycopene prevents oxidation of LDL cholesterol and reduces the risk of developing atherosclerosis and coronary disease. In addition, it can reduce the risk of prostate cancer and cancers of the lung, bladder, cervix, and skin. The most compelling evidence so far for its effectiveness is the role of lycopene in prostate cancer prevention (327–336).

N

N-acetyl Cysteine

N-acetyl cysteine (NAC) is a derivative of the protein amino acid L-cysteine. NAC has antioxidant activity and also may be converted to L-cysteine in the body, which in turn may be used to form the antioxidant glutathione. Glutathione is a potent antioxidant and important for healthy immune function. NAC may play a role in benefiting liver and heart health, immune function, and pulmonary and respiratory problems.

O

Omega-3 Fatty Acids

Omega-3 fatty acids are long-chain polyunsaturated fatty acids. The fish-based and fish-oil-based omega-3 fatty acids consist of EPA (twenty carbon atoms) and DHA (twenty-two carbon atoms). Plant foods and vegetable oils lack EPA and DHA, but some do contain varying amounts of alpha-linolenic acid (eighteen carbon atoms). Diets rich in omega-3 fatty acids may help lower blood triglycerides and increase HDL cholesterol. Omega-3 fatty acids may also act as an anticoagulant to prevent blood from clotting. Several other studies also suggest that these fatty acids may also help lower high blood pressure (337–340). Many vegetable oils are greatly enriched in omega-6 fatty acids (mainly as linoleic acid in corn, safflower, sunflower, and soybean oils).

P

Phenols

Phenols—also known as phenolic compounds—are natural chemicals found in most plant products but are richly concentrated in fruit, wine, tea, and chocolate. These substances give the taste of bitterness or astringency. This sharp and biting flavor is evident in dry red wine, baking or cooking chocolate, black coffee, or unripe persimmons. This somewhat unfavorable characteristic can be made inconspicuous when sugar is added.

Proanthocyanidins Oligomers (PCO) (see Grapeseed Extract)

O

Oligomeric Proanthocyanidins (OPC) (see Grapeseed Extract)

S

Selenium

Selenium is a trace mineral found in soil. It comes in several forms, and only minute quantities of it are needed, although the lack of it can cause many problems in the human body. Selenium becomes part of nearly every cell, with particularly high concentrations in the kidneys, liver, pancreas, spleen, and testes. The dietary sources for selenium are usually associated with the soil in which the food was grown. Vegetables and grain products often have higher selenium contents if they are grown in soil rich in selenium content. The most concentrated food source for selenium is the Brazil nut; a single one contains 120 mcg. Seafood in general, as well as poultry and meat, are also good sources. So are grains, especially oats and brown rice. Dairy products are also an excellent dietary source of selenium.

Selenium's primary function in the human body is to work in conjunction with vitamin E. It is also necessary in the slowing of the aging process. The prostoglandins in the human body, which protect against high blood pressure, cannot be formed without selenium. Because it boosts the body's antioxidant capacity, selenium is thought to have some ability to control cell damage that may lead to cancer. In addition, selenium may even act in other ways to stop early cancer by (1) boosting the immune system and fighting off infection and cancer cells, (2) retarding the effects of aging, (3) protecting against heart attack and stroke, and (4) guarding against cataracts and macular degeneration.

T

Turmeric

Turmeric is an spice used since antiquity as a dye and a condiment. It is a member of the ginger family. Like ginger, it is the root of the turmeric plant that is used as a spice, usually in a dried form. Turmeric contains compounds called curcuminoids, which are very strong antioxidants. Curcuminoids may have anti-cancer and anti-inflammatory benefits. Some research indicates they may also have antiviral and antifungal benefits and possibly protect against atherosclerosis (341–352).

V

Vitamins

The term vitamin is derived from the words vital and amine, because vitamins are required for life and were originally thought to be amines—a class of organic compounds with a certain chemical structure. Interestingly, not all vitamins are amines; however, they are organic compounds required by humans in small amounts from the diet. Therefore, any organic compound is considered a vitamin if a lack of that compound in the diet results in overt symptoms of deficiency (594).

Vitamin A

Vitamin A is a generic term for a large number of related compounds. Retinol and retinal are preformed vitamin A. Vitamin A is a family of fat-soluble vitamins. Retinol is one of the most active forms of vitamin A and is found in liver and eggs. Retinol is called pro-vitamin A. It can be converted to retinal and retinoic acid, the active forms of vitamin A. Beta-carotene is a pro-vitamin A carotenoids that is more competently converted to retinol than other carotenoids (595–604).

Some plant foods contain darkly colored pigments called pro-vitamin A carotenoids that can be converted to vitamin A.

Vitamin A plays an important role in vision, bone growth, reproduction, cell division, and cell differentiation. It also helps maintain the surface linings of the eyes and the respiratory, urinary, and intestinal tracts, and maintains the integrity of skin and mucous membranes that function as a barrier to bacteria and viruses. Vitamin A and some carotenoids regulate the immune system and also act as an antioxidant (594).

The Recommended Dietary Allowance (RDA)

The RDA for vitamin A is based on the amount needed to ensure adequate stores of vitamin A for four months to support normal reproductive function, immune function, gene expression, and vision (595–594). This is equal to 700–900 mcg/day or 2,500–3,000 IU/day.

Vitamin B-Complex

Biotin

Biotin is a water-soluble vitamin that is classified as a B-complex vitamin. Biotin is required by all organisms but can be synthesized only by bacteria, yeasts, algae, and some plant species (558–559). Biotin is an integral part of special mammalian enzymes known as carboxylases, of which there are five types (560). These five different carboxylases facilitate essential metabolic reaction involved in synthesis and metabolism of fatty acids, formation of glucose from sources other than carbohydrates and starches (e.g. amino acids), catabolism of leucine which is an essential amino acid, and synthesis of some other complex and unique molecules such as odd chain fatty acids and certain amino acids. Lastly, addition of the biotin on the proteins that surround the DNA—the histones—plays a role in regulating DNA replication and transcription as well as cellular proliferation (560–565).

The Adequate Intake (AI)

Due to insufficient clinical evidence to calculate a RDA for biotin, the AI for biotin is 35 mcg to 60 mcg/day (557–558).

Folic Acid

Folic acid (folate) is a water-soluble B-complex vitamin. Folic acid occurs rarely in foods or your body but due to its stability is often used in vitamin supplements and fortified foods. Naturally occurring folates exist in many chemical forms and are found in foods as well as in metabolically active forms in the human body (1). The only function of folic acid in your body is to facilitate the transfer of one-carbon units (2). Folic acid acts as acceptor and donor of one-carbon units in a variety of reactions essential for the metabolism of nucleic acids and amino acids (3). In addition, folic acid is required for the synthesis of methionine which is integral and necessary for the synthesis of S-adenosylmethionine (SAM). SAM is the donor of the one-carbon unit known as a methyl group (used in many biological reactions, including methylation of DNA, which may be important in cancer prevention). Additionally, folic acid is required for the metabolism of several important amino acids. For example, the synthesis of methionine from homocysteine requires folic acid as well as vitamin B12. Hence, folic acid deficiency can result in decreased synthesis of methionine and a buildup of homocysteine which may be a risk factor for heart disease as well as several other chronic diseases

Riboflavin (Vitamin B2)

Riboflavin (Vitamin B2) is a water-soluble B vitamin. It is the central and integral component of a special compounds called FAD and FMN (576–585). These compounds are another group of molecules that all living organisms use during metabolic reactions. These metabolic reactions are involved in capturing and donating energy from digestion of food. FAD is part of the electron transport (respiratory) chain, which is central to energy production. Both FAD and FMN participate in redox reactions in numerous metabolic pathways (578, 579). These enzymes are critical for the metabolism of carbohydrates, fats, and proteins and also critical in the metabolism of variety of drugs and toxins (4). Another important function of these essential compounds are the central role that they play glutathione redox cycle plays a major role in removing harmful molecules generated from reactive oxygen species, thereby protecting organisms. Additionally, xanthine oxidase, another FAD-dependent enzyme, is involved in uric acid metabolism. Uric acid is one of the most effective water-soluble antioxidants in the blood. Riboflavin deficiency can result in decreased xanthine oxidase activity, reducing blood uric acid levels (582, 583).

The Recommended Dietary Allowance (RDA)

The RDA for riboflavin is based on the prevention of deficiency. Clinical signs of deficiency in humans appear at intakes of less than 0.5 milligrams (mg)/day, and intake of 1 mg/day is recommended (576).

Niacin (Vitamin B3)

Niacin also known as nicotinic acid or vitamin B3 is a water-soluble vitamin. Niacin, is used by your body to form two very important compounds called NAD and NADP (567–575). These two compounds are vital and required by more than two hundred enzymes in your body that are involved in metabolic, anabolic, and catabolic reactions. NAD and NADP act mainly either to accept or donate electrons for reactions in energy-producing and energy-requiring reactions. All living organisms derive most of their energy from oxidation-reduction reactions, which are processes involving the transfer of electrons with both NAD and NADP as central components of these reactions. Without them, no food can be used as energy by your body! For example, NAD is involved in catabolism or degradation of carbohydrates, fats, proteins, and alcohol. On the other hand NADP functions more often in biosynthetic and anabolic reactions, such as in the synthesis of complex molecules including fatty acids and cholesterol (566, 567).

The RDA for niacin, is based on the prevention of deficiency. Many niacin deficiencies can be prevented with intake of about 15 mg/day (569–575)

Vitamin B5 (Pantothenic Acid)

Pantothenic acid, also known as vitamin B5, is essential to all living organisms (550–555). Pantothenic acid is found throughout living cells in the form of coenzyme A (CoA), a vital compound essential in numerous chemical reactions in the cells of your body that are necessary to sustain life! Coenzyme A is required for chemical reactions that convert fat, carbohydrates, and proteins to energy. Coenzyme A, through a chemical reaction known as acetylation reaction, modifies important proteins in your body by the addition of an acetate group that is donated by the CoA molecules. These modified acetylated proteins play a major role in the cell division and DNA replication. In addition, a carrier called acyl-carrier protein is essential for fatty acid synthesis. The acyl-carrier protein requires pantothenic acid (554, 555). Both CoA and the acyl-carrier protein are required for the synthesis of fatty acids, which are an integral part of all cell membranes and nerve sheaths.

The synthesis of a variety of important and vital molecules, such as essential fats, cholesterol, and steroid hormones, requires CoA, as well as the synthesis of the neurotransmitter acetylcholine and the hormone, melatonin. Other important cell pathways that require CoA are the synthesis of heme, which is the central component of hemoglobin, and also other pathways related to metabolism of a variety of drugs and toxins by the liver (552, 553).

The Adequate Intake (AI)

The AI for pantothenic acid is based on estimated dietary intakes in healthy adult population groups which is about 5 mg/day (557).

Vitamin B6

Vitamin B6 is a water-soluble vitamin also known as pyridoxine which has a great importance in human metabolism (518–533). Vitamin B6 must be obtained from your diet since your body cannot synthesize it. Amazingly, vitamin B6 plays a vital role in the function of more than one hundred enzymes that facilitate essential chemical reactions in your body (518–523). Vitamin B6 is required for the following (1) proper nervous system function, (2) formation and proper function of red blood cells, (3) synthesis of another important vitamin B type called niacin, (4) synthesis and improvement of hormone function, and last but not least (5) synthesis of nucleic acid for DNA and RNA production.

Deficiency

Severe deficiency of vitamin B6 is uncommon. Alcoholics are thought to be most at risk of vitamin B6 deficiency due to low dietary intakes and impaired metabolism of the vitamin.

The recommended dietary allowance (RDA) is about 1.5–2.0 mg/day. However, because vitamin B6 is involved in many aspects of metabolism, several factors may increase your requirement for vitamin B6. Of those factors, protein intake has been the most studied. If you increase your dietary protein, your requirement for vitamin B6 is also increases, probably because vitamin B6 is a required compound for many enzymes involved in amino acid metabolism (524).

Vitamin B12 (Cobalamin)

Vitamin B12, also known as cobalamin, is a unique vitamin since it not only has the largest and most complex chemical structure of all the vitamins, but also it is the only vitamin that contains a metal ion, cobalt (586–590). The cobalamin is a cofactor for only two essential and vital enzymes called methionine synthase and L-methylmalonyl-CoA mutase (587). These compounds are required for the synthesis of the amino acid methionine from homocysteine. Methionine in turn is required for the synthesis of a methyl group donor called S-adenosylmethionineb (SAM), which is extensively in methylation of important sites within DNA and RNA (588). This methylation of DNA is very important in cancer prevention. Furthermore, inadequate function of these vital compounds can also lead to an accumulation of homocysteine, which has been associated with increased risk of cardiovascular diseases.

The current RDA is about 2.5 mcg/day. However, due to the increased risk of food-bound vitamin B12 malabsorption in older adults, it is recommended that adults over fifty years of age get most of the RDA from fortified food or vitamin B12–containing supplements (592).

Vitamin C

Vitamin C (ascorbic acid) is a water-soluble vitamin that, in spite of its amazing properties, your body does not have the ability to produce! Therefore, you must provide your body with vitamin C through ingestion of food containing this essential vitamin.

Vitamin C is a well-known and highly prized and extremely effective antioxidant. Amazingly, even at low tissue levels, it can protect many vital molecules in your body, such as DNA, RNA, lipids, proteins, and cell membranes. This vitamin is a regarded as the potent scavenger of the notorious free radicals and reactive oxygen species that are detrimental to your body and ultimately your health (508–517). These free radicals and reactive oxygen species are generated as a by-product of normal metabolism in your body. In addition, they can also be generated as a consequence of exposure to environmental pollutants and toxins. Still more, this vitamin has the unusual ability to recharge/regenerate other antioxidants, such as vitamin E. For example, it has been shown that the oxidized form of the vitamin E can be regenerated by vitamin C (508).

Briefly, vitamin C is essential for the proper synthesis of collagen, which is an important structural component of many body tissues and organs, such as blood vessels, tendons, and bones. Besides, vitamin C is critical for several other important organ functions in your body. Vitamin C is indispensable for proper brain function, since it plays a vital role in the synthesis of the special neurotransmitter norepinephrine. Neurotransmitters are chemicals produced in the neurons that are required for different parts of the body to communicate and function (508–517).

Another important function of vitamin C is that it is required for the synthesis of carnitine, which is a small molecule that is paramount for the transport of fat into special components of the mitochondria cells, where it is converted to energy. Some clinical research advocates that vitamin C is involved in the metabolism of cholesterol to bile acids, which may be used to lower your blood cholesterol levels, as well as the incidence of gallstones.

Vitamin C, also known as ascorbic acid, plays an integral role in the human body in many enzymatic functions as well as being vital for the proper growth and development of teeth, bones, gums, and blood vessels. In fact, vitamin C is a component in all the organs in the human body. In addition, without vitamin C, your body would not be able to absorb two important substances: iron and folic acid.

Furthermore, vitamin C is an antioxidant that can help neutralize many free radicals, thereby playing a protective role against toxic compounds formed from oxidized lipids and preventing the genetic damage or inflammation they can cause.

Vitamin C is found in most fruits and vegetables, with citrus fruits having the highest concentrations of this vitamin. You can get your dietary vitamin C through many vegetables, including tomatoes and green leafy vegetables and such fruits as cantaloupe, honeydew, and strawberries.

In the United States, the RDA for vitamin C is approximately 100 mg/day. The recommended intake for smokers is 35 mg/day higher than for nonsmokers, since they have lower vitamin C level and higher oxidative stress due to the toxins in cigarette smoke (514).

Vitamin D

Vitamin D is a fat-soluble vitamin that is essential for many cells as well as maintaining normal calcium metabolism (534). Vitamin D is truly a hormone that is essential for proper function of the cells in your body. Vitamin D is considered a hormone, since it has a specific receptor within the cell nucleus! Vitamin D3 (cholecalciferol) can be synthesized in your skin upon exposure to ultraviolet-B (UVB) radiation from sunlight. It can also be absorbed by your body from the diet. Plants synthesize a weaker form of the vitamin D called ergosterol, which is converted to vitamin D2 (ergocalciferol) by ultraviolet light. Since the production of vitamin D in your skin is not sufficient, adequate intake of vitamin D from the diet is essential for health.

Interestingly, vitamin D is biologically inactive, and it must be converted to its biologically active forms, first by the liver and then by the kidneys.

Most of the physiological effects of vitamin D in your body are related to the activity of the highly potent 1,25 dihydroxy vitamin D that is generated in the kidneys (535–538). As mentioned before, the majority of the biological effects of vitamin D are mediated through the vitamin D receptor (VDR) in the cell nucleus (538). Upon entering the nucleus of a cell, vitamin D initiates a cascade of molecular interactions that modulate the activation of more than fifty genes in the tissues throughout your body (539).

Maintenance of serum calcium levels within a narrow range is vital for normal functioning of the nervous system, as well as for bone growth and maintenance of bone density. Vitamin D is essential for the efficient utilization of calcium by the body (534). In addition, it is vital for cell differentiation and specialization to proper cells in your body for adequate immunity, since vitamin D is a potent immune system modulator. Additionally, it is required for proper insulin secretion and blood pressure regulation.

The Adequate Intake (AI)

Due to variable factors that can affect the vitamin D requirement (sunlight exposure), it impossible to calculate an RDA (543). Thus, many experts believe that the adequate intake levels should be increased due to the importance of this vital vitamin. Therefore, the American Academy of Pediatrics has increased their vitamin D intake recommendation to 400 IU/day for all infants, children, and adolescents (544). Still, there is plenty of research that supports intake of as high as 1,000 IU/day (545–549).

Vitamin E

Vitamin E is part of a group of substances called tocopherol. It is a fat-soluble vitamin that exists in as many as eight different forms, each with its own biological activity. Alpha-tocopherol (α-tocopherol) is the name of the most active form of vitamin E in humans. It is also a powerful antioxidant. The synthetic form of this vitamin is only half as active as the natural form.

Because it is fat soluble, vitamin E it can be stored in body fat. Its protective role has been widely studied. Since it has strong antioxidant properties, it may protect against heart disease and cancer. Vitamin E has also been shown to play a role in the immune function, in DNA repair, and other metabolic processes.

Vitamin E is found in the fatty parts of foods. The best sources of vitamin E are vegetable oils, such as sunflower, safflower, canola, olive, and wheat-germ oils. It is also found in avocados, nuts, seeds, wheat germ, and whole-grain (unrefined) products. Green leafy vegetables have smaller amounts.

Z

Zeaxanthin

Lutein and zeaxanthin are two antioxidants found highly concentrated in the macula. They give the macula its characteristic yellow appearance. Zeaxanthin and lutein are strongly associated with a reduced risk of cataracts and macular degeneration. Zeaxanthin cannot be synthesized by humans and must be obtained from the diet. It is obtained primarily from dark green leafy vegetables, such as spinach, collard greens, kale, mustard greens, and turnip greens.

Some Antioxidants:

Name of Antioxidant	Sources of Antioxidant
Beta-carotene	All colorful fruits and vegetables, carrots, kale, parsley, spinach, turnips, apricots, peaches
Coenzyme Q10	Organ meats (especially hearts) are the richest sources. Beef and chicken contain smaller amounts.
Ellagic acid	Berries, pecans, walnuts, pomegranates
Hesperidin	Oranges, tangelos, lemons
Lutein	Corn, egg yolks, and green vegetables and fruits, broccoli, brussels sprouts, kale, cabbage, green beans, green peas, spinach, kiwifruit, and honeydew melon
Lycopene	Tomatoes, watermelon, papaya, pink grapefruit, and pink guava

N-acetyl cysteine	No dietary source
Proanthocyanidins	Grape seeds
Quercetin	Onions, green tea, and red wine
Selenium	Seafood, meat, grains and seeds
Turmeric	Turmeric, curry
Vitamin E	Unprocessed vegetable oils, whole grains, dark green leafy vegetables, nuts, and legumes
Vitamin C	Oranges, grapefruits, tangerines, berries, broccoli, brussels sprouts, collards, guava, kale, turnip greens, sweet peppers, cabbage, cauliflower, spinach, watercress, melon
Zeaxanthin	Egg yolk, vegetables

List of Food Sources of Powerful Antioxidants

Animal Products

Eggs
Fish
Liver
Shellfish

Cereals

Barley
Corn
Flaxseed
Millet
Oatmeal Oats
Rye
Soy
Whole grains

Fruits

Apricots
Black currants
Blueberries

Cantaloupe
Cherries
Citrus fruits
Cranberries
Dates
Grapefruit
Grapes
Kiwifruit
Lemons
Limes
Oranges
Peaches
Pineapple
Pink grapefruit
Plums
Pomegranates
Prunes
Raisins
Raspberries
Red grapes (Red wine)
Sour cherries
Strawberries
Watermelon

Legumes

All types of beans
Nuts
Soybeans

Nuts, Seeds

Alfalfa
All types of seeds
Almonds
Brazil nuts
Cashews
Hazelnuts

Macadamia nuts
Sunflower seeds
Walnuts

Vegetables

Artichokes
Beets
Broccoli
Brussels sprouts
Carrots
Chili peppers
Collards
Corn
Eggplant
Green leafy vegetables
Green peppers
Kale
Onions
Parsley
Peppers
Red bell peppers
Red cabbage
Spinach
Squash
Sweet potatoes
Tomato products
Tomatoes

Roots and Tubers

Ginger
Tumeric

Name of the Major Known Antioxidants and Their Food Sources

Beta-carotene: All colorful fruits and vegetables, carrots, kale, parsley, spinach, turnips, apricots, peaches

Coenzyme Q10: Organ meats (especially hearts) are the richest sources. Beef and chicken contain smaller amounts.

Ellagic acid: Berries, pecans, walnuts, pomegranates

Glutathione: Asparagus, broccoli, avocado garlic, and spinach are also known to boost glutathione levels. In addition fresh unprocessed meats contain high levels of sulphur-containing amino acids and help to maintain optimal glutathione levels.

Hesperidin: Oranges, tangelos, lemons

Lignan: Flax seed, oatmeal, barley, rye

Lutein: Corn, egg yolks, green vegetables and fruits, broccoli, Brussels sprouts, kale, cabbage, green beans, green peas, spinach, kiwifruit, honeydew melon

Lycopene: Tomatoes, tomato products, pink grapefruit, watermelon, papaya, pink guava

Phytochemicals and Flavonoids/polyphenols: red wine, soy, red grapes, cranberries

Proanthocyanidins: Grape seeds

Quercetin: Onions, green tea, red wine

Selenium: Fish, shellfish, red meat, grains, eggs, chicken, garlic, seeds

Turmeric: Turmeric, curry

Vitamin A and Carotenoids: Carrots, squash, broccoli, sweet potatoes, tomatoes, kale, collards, cantaloupe, peaches, and apricots (brightly colored fruits and vegetables)

Vitamin C: Oranges, grapefruits, tangerines, berries, broccoli, Brussels sprouts, collards, guava, kale, turnip greens, sweet peppers, cabbage, cauliflower, spinach, watercress, melons

Vitamin E: Unprocessed vegetable oils, whole grains, dark green leafy vegetables, nuts, and legumes.

Zeaxanthin: Egg yolks, vegetables, green beans, green peas

Note: Fruit drinks, cocktails, or punches do not count as real fruit juices. Check the label for 100 percent juice. If fresh vegetables and fruit are not in season, frozen or dried fruits and vegetables are just as healthy. However, most canned foods are salted and may not be equal to fresh fruits and vegetables in quality.

List of Fruits with Highest ORAC (Units per 100 grams)

Prunes	5,770
Raisins	2,830
Blueberries	2,400
Blackberries	2,036
Strawberries	1,540
Raspberries	1,220
Plums	949
Oranges	750
Red grapes	739
Cherries	670

List of Vegetables with Highest ORAC (Units per 100 grams)

Kale	1,770
Spinach	1,260
Brussels sprouts	980
Alfalfa sprouts	930
Broccoli florets	890
Beets	840
Red bell peppers	710
Onions	450

Corn	400
Eggplant	390

Benefits of Vegetables and Fruits

+ Excellent source of carbohydrates with low-Glycemic Index ratings

+ Excellent source of vitamins and minerals

+ High in fiber

+ Low in fat and calories

+ Rich in antioxidants

+ Rich in phytochemicals

Beta-carotene	In orange-colored foods like sweet potatoes, carrots, squash, pumpkins, mangoes. Also in some green leafy vegetables like spinach, kale.
Lutein	In green leafy vegetables like collard greens, spinach, kale.
Lycopene	In tomatoes, watermelon, guava, papaya, apricots, pink grapefruit.
Vitamin A	In liver, sweet potatoes, carrots, milk, egg yolks.
Vitamin C	In many vegetables and fruits, cereals, poultry, fish.
Vitamin E	In almonds and other nuts, many oils such as safflower, corn, and soybean. Also in mangoes, Swiss chard, and sweet potatoes.
Selenium	In rice, wheat, Brazil nuts.

A daily recommended antioxidant intake has not been established. However, eight to ten daily servings of fruits and vegetables—which is equivalent to four thousand to seven thousand ORAC units—should be taken daily.

A Good-Tasting Antioxidant: Chocolate

Chocolate is a complex and exciting food, which has several effects on human behavior. There is something in chocolate that affects the chemistry of the brain in the same manner as love—thus, we often substitute chocolate for love, or give chocolates when we feel in love. For these and many other reasons, researchers and scientists have explored the chemical ingredients in chocolate in order to unlock its secrets. Chocolate contains, among a number of chemicals, two particular substances, phenylethylamine and serotonin, both of which are brain chemicals that elevate your mood. Chocolate is good for your mental health.

These mood-lifting chemicals, which are produced naturally in your brain, are released when you feel happy or in love. Increased levels of serotonin also alleviate depression. Eating chocolate causes a release of these agents in the brain that provides a boost when you are feeling sad or depressed. Chocolate also releases endorphins, natural opiate-like substances in the brain that reduce pain.

Clinical studies show that chocolate, in moderation, is actually good for you. It may prevent heart disease, cancer, and other degenerative illnesses (353–357).

Cocoa beans and chocolate contain several potent antioxidants, such as catechins and phenols. These particular antioxidants play a pivotal role in the prevention of diseases such as cancer and heart disease. Catechins can also be found in fruits and vegetables and tea. However, chocolate, particularly dark chocolate, is a good source of catechins, and it contains a significantly greater amount than tea—up to four times more.

On average, dark chocolate contains 50 percent fat. Stearic acid, which is the chief source of saturated fat in chocolate, seems to have no effect on blood cholesterol levels (358–370).

Chocolate, like red wine, contains a class of strong antioxidants called phenols. Phenols are said to prevent LDL cholesterols in your bloodstream from oxidizing and clogging your major arteries and coronaries by the development of atherosclerosis. Atherosclerosis is the process by which plaque forms in the walls of arteries supplying your major organs, depositing oxidized LDL, which can lead to disease.

A word of caution: chocolate is high in calories, and eating too much can make you fat. Therefore, the overeating of chocolate can lead to obesity.

Chocolate also contains essential nutrients, such as iron, calcium, and potassium, and vitamins A, B1, C, D, and E.

As mentioned before, chocolate contains a lot of phenylethylamine, which makes people feel as though they're in love. As soon as you consume chocolate, it releases phenylethylamine and serotonin into your brain, producing the same arousing effects as when you experience a feeling of passion, love, or lust. Despite scientific difficulty in proving chocolate is an aphrodisiac, it does contain substances that increase energy, stamina, and feelings of well-being.

The reality is that chocolate makes you feel good and induces feelings of being in love. Perhaps these noticeable effects have given chocolate its famous reputation as an aphrodisiac.

The Darker the Chocolate, the Better It Is

The different forms of chocolate are as follows:

+ Unsweetened chocolate for baking is a mixture of cocoa powder and refined cocoa butter. It is too bitter to eat.

+ Dark chocolate contains cocoa, cocoa butter, and varying amounts of sugar.

+ Milk chocolate has milk as well as cocoa, cocoa butter, and varying amounts of sugar.

+ White chocolate contains no chocolate and no polyphenols, only cocoa butter, sugar, milk, and flavorings.

Choosing High Antioxidant Foods

Always choose foods with high ORAC values. Your total intake should be between three thousand and four thousand ORAC units, which translates to ten servings of fruits and vegetables per day. Choices include five fruit and five vegetable selections. Eating ten servings of fruits and vegetables per day should provide an ORAC intake of thirty-three hundred to thirty-five hundred units.

High ORAC value fruits are generally strongly colored. The foods with the blue, reddish, and dark green hues have the highest ORAC values and offer the most protection.

Certain fruit juices can be substitutes for one high ORAC value fruit. Twelve ounces of the following juices can substitute for one high ORAC fruit serving:

Cherry juice
Cranberry juice
Grape juice
Orange juice
Pomegranate juice
Blueberry juice

(Do not substitute for more than one fruit.)

ORAC Value of Common Fruits and Vegetables: Whole Fruit, Not Juice
ORAC units per 100-grams/3.5 oz.

Alfalfa Sprouts	930
Apple	207
Apricot	175
Banana	210
Beets	840
Blackberries	2,036
Blueberries	2,400
Broccoli Florets	890
Brussels Sprouts	980
Cabbage	295
Cantaloupe	250
Carrot	200
Cauliflower	385
Celery	75
Cherries	670
Corn	400

Cucumber	60
Dark Chocolate	13,120
Eggplant	390
Grapes, red	739
Grapes, white	460
Honeydew Melon	97
Head Lettuce	105
Kale	1,770
Kiwifruit	610
Leaf Lettuce	265
Milk Chocolate	6,740
Onion	450
Oranges	750
Peach	170
Pear	110
Peas, Frozen	375
Pink Grapefruit	495
Plums	949
Potato	300
Prunes	5,770
Raisins	2,830
Raspberries	1,220
Red Bell Pepper	710
Red grapes	739
Spinach	1,260
Sprouts	980
Strawberries	1,540
String Beans	200
Sweet Potato	295
Tofu	205
Tomato	195
Watermelon	100
Yellow Squash	150

Chapter Nine

Detoxification

Detoxification is a method to remove harmful chemicals and toxins from your body. A detoxification diet (detox diet) is a natural way to achieve this goal. The human body is equipped with three major organs that carry out this major and significant task: the kidneys, liver, and colon. These organs detoxify and excrete most of the toxins ingested or produced through metabolism. The organs can be overwhelmed if the amount of toxins surpasses their ability to detox. As a result, harmful toxins accumulate and build up in your body and can cause wide-ranging problems, from tiredness and headaches to weight gain and acne. Using a proper cleansing system, you can help your body do a more complete job of the purifying and purging of toxins.

Organs Involved in Body Detoxification

Excretion is the process of removing harmful and toxic substances formed in the body. These substances, usually nitrogenous substances such as urea, are usually waste materials produced by complex chemical reactions taking place in every living cell as part of metabolism. As part of the metabolism of nutrients ingested, waste products and toxins are formed that need to be excreted, otherwise they will lead to an accumulation of these products, which can adversely affect your health.

The three major organs involved are:

+ Liver
+ Colon
+ Kidneys

Each of these organs has a specific function in ridding your body rid of unwanted substances and metabolites. They work in concert help your body to detoxify daily, hourly, and every minute.

Colon, liver, and kidney diseases can have a devastating effect on how your body functions. Proper nutrition and appropriate care of these organs are extremely important.

The Liver—A Detoxification Organ

The liver is a very complex and important organ in your body; it performs over five hundred essential functions. The two major functions of the liver are detoxification and control of amino acid metabolism.

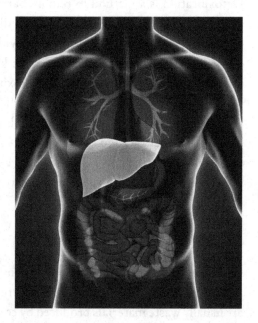

Ammonium, bilirubin, and urea are the three major toxins produced in the liver. They are by-products of amino acid and hemoglobin breakdown. Interestingly, your body may use some of these compounds in the production of nitrogen compounds. For example, ammonium ions can be converted to urea.

Ammonium and Urea

Your body is unable to store proteins or amino acids—the building blocks of proteins. When you ingest large amounts of protein, the excess amino acids produced from digesting proteins are transported to the liver from your intestine. Your liver cells perform several complicated actions on the absorbed amino acids, converting them into ammonia. However, through further actions, your liver converts the non-nitrogenous portions of the amino acids to carbohydrates or fats.

Ammonia is highly toxic in the body and, therefore, cannot be allowed to accumulate. Through several important actions, the liver converts the ammonia molecule to the less toxic compound urea.

Urea is released into the bloodstream and excreted by your kidneys. Your kidneys filter the urea, which is removed from your body in the form of urine.

Bilirubin

Another important and clinically relevant example of waste elimination by the liver is bilirubin, the toxic breakdown product of hemoglobin in the red blood cells. As red blood cells age or become damaged, they have to be eliminated from blood circulation. Your liver accomplishes this major task. Due to the large numbers of red blood cells in your body, bilirubin is generated in large quantities every day. For example, every minute, almost twenty million of your red blood cells are taken out of circulation and are disposed. These fragile, aged, and damaged red blood cells are picked up by special cells in your liver and other parts of your body and are digested.

The hemoglobin liberated from these red cells is converted into bilirubin, which is excreted as bile into your gut. Also, bile consists of many compounds and toxins, such as endogenous molecules (steroids, hormones) and exogenous compounds (antibiotics and metabolites of drugs). A substantial number of these compounds are reabsorbed in the small intestine and ultimately eliminated by the kidney.

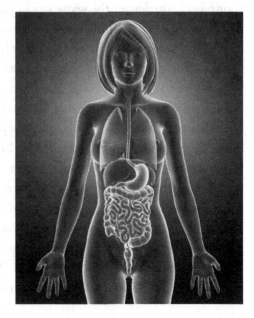

The Colon–A Detoxification Organ

Another very important and vital organ in detoxification of your body is the large intestine, otherwise known as the colon. Your colon is intended to function as a smoothly flowing system to promptly flush digestive wastes from your body. The colon can be viewed as the conduit by which your body gets rid of waste products that are formed during the digestive processes.

If this cleansing process is halted, it can cause many symptoms and ailments. Over ninety-five million Americans experience some kind of digestive problem. Over ten million people are hospitalized each year for care of gastrointestinal problems. Even though many digestive problems are more common in older people, they can occur at any age, even in children. Interestingly, according to the American College of Gastroenterology, all Americans are susceptible to digestive problems, regardless of gender, ethnic, or socioeconomic backgrounds (371, 372).

Regular bowel movements are important for your optimal health. Some believe that if you don't have at least one bowel movement per day, you are not getting toxins out of your system promptly. Even though our bowel physiology has remained the same for many centuries, our diet has changed drastically. So, it is no surprise that colon cancer is the second-leading cause of cancer deaths in the United States.

In our society, the most frequent bowel problem people experience is constipation. As a consequence of constipation, the transition time of toxic wastes is very slow. It is evident that the longer it takes to excrete the waste—"transit time"—the longer your body is exposed to the toxic waste matter in your bowel. The longer the waste sits in your colon, the greater the risk of developing disease. So, infrequent bowel movements over an extended period of time may be hazardous to your health. It is a good idea to avoid constipating foods and increase the rate of waste removal naturally by ingesting more fiber. This will lead to a regular bowel movement, which cleanses the bowel.

Furthermore, a properly functioning colon is necessary for the transport of nutrients. The lining of the colon is very important in the absorption of minerals and water and in eliminating body wastes from the system. If your colon has accumulated feces, it cannot absorb nutrients or eliminate wastes properly. A segment of the population may require temporary help in battling constipation. There are many over-the-counter laxatives available, but these laxatives can be quite dangerous. Many physicians, including gastroenterologists, believe in simple, natural, and gentle colon cleansing. This can be achieved with increasing high-fiber fruits and vegetables in your diet combined with increasing your water intake throughout the day.

The Kidney—A Detoxification Organ

Most people are born with two kidneys. Your kidneys are bean-shaped organs, each approximately the size of your clenched fist. They are located in your flanks, on each side of your body. Understanding how your kidneys work can help to keep them healthy. Your kidneys filter your blood to remove waste products, such as urea, creatinine, and numerous other toxins.

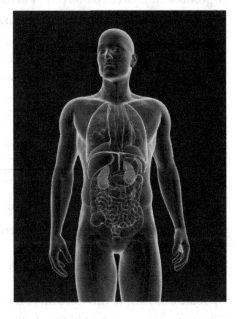

The kidneys are another group of sophisticated detoxifying machines. However, your two kidneys are vital organs that perform many functions, including hormone production to maintain your bones and your red blood cell production. They help maintain body water and regulate your blood pressure. In addition, they detoxify your blood and maintain its narrow and essential chemical balance. The kidneys also remove wastes and extra water from the blood via urine.

Each of your kidneys is made up of approximately one million filtering units called nephrons. Your kidneys filter and process approximately fifty gallons of your blood daily via these nephrons. Then, this filtered blood is processed in many ways to excrete about half a gallon of waste products and extra water as urine. This is a remarkable feat.

As mentioned previously, the waste products and toxins in your blood are formed from the normal metabolism and breakdown of tissues and food you eat. Your body uses the food for energy and self-repair. After your body has taken what it needs from the food, waste is sent to the blood.

If your kidneys fail to remove these waste products, they will build up in the blood and damage your body. The buildup of waste products, including urea in the body, results in uremia. Uremia affects all the systems in the body and can make you feel quite ill. If uremia is not treated, you may develop symptoms such as headache, nausea, vomiting, poor appetite, extreme fatigue, and mental cloudiness.

Also, your kidneys maintain and regulate a tight level of important substances and chemicals like sodium, bicarbonate, magnesium, calcium, phosphorus, and potassium. As your kidneys fail, your body may not be able to produce enough red blood cells. Furthermore, your blood chemistry—the right balance of chemicals such as potassium, calcium, and phosphorous—may become abnormal.

Several Important Functions of Kidneys

Kidneys maintain water balance—Remove excess water
Renin—Maintains blood pressure
Calcitriol—Maintains healthy bones
Erythropoietin—Signals production of red blood cells
Kidneys maintain normal blood chemistry—Maintain electrolytes
Kidneys remove waste products—Detoxify blood

Kidney Disease

By some estimation, there are more than twenty million people with some form of early or moderate kidney failure (25, 26). The most common causes of kidney disease and heart disease are diabetes and high blood pressure.

Major Causes of Kidney Failure

+ Inflammation of the kidneys (glomerulonephritis)
+ Diabetes
+ High blood pressure
+ Arteriosclerosis
+ Obstructions of urinary system
+ Toxins
+ Herbal medicines
+ Medications
+ Polycystic kidney disease

+ Infection

+ Kidney stones

+ Physical injury

Severe infections, drugs, poisons, physical injury, or blockage can also lead to kidney failure. As kidneys lose the ability to function, toxins and waste products accumulate in your body. This will lead to an accumulation of water and harmful metabolites and toxins like uric acid, urea, and lactic acid. As a result of this buildup of toxins and water, you will start to feel tired and sick. This buildup is called uremia.

Interestingly, even if you have kidney failure, you will probably keep urinating the same amount. Even though you urinate the same volume as before, the amount of waste products in the urine is low and will continue to build up in the blood. A simple blood test measuring creatinine and urea can demonstrate if you have a kidney problem. Unfortunately, many doctors may miss early kidney disease that only shows a mild increase in urea and creatinine.

Kidney disease advances in stages, and its early stages fail to show any obvious signs or symptoms. As your kidneys stop working, you may feel certain symptoms, such as:

+ Extreme fatigue

+ Nausea and vomiting

+ Shortness of breath

+ Difficulty sleeping

+ Swelling in the hands, face, feet, and body

+ Loss of appetite

+ Bad taste in the mouth

+ Bad odor in the mouth

+ Urinating often at night (during sleep, must wake up and urinate, often several times)

+ Itchiness

+ High blood pressure

The earlier you are diagnosed with kidney disease, the sooner you can start therapy and the better your chances of controlling its progression. Nutrition, diet, control of blood pressure, salt and protein restriction, control of blood sugar, and medications are important treatments for kidney failure. The diet for the early stages of kidney failure is intended to minimize the amount of waste products in the blood, which will decrease the work of the kidneys. Controlling the amount of protein, phosphorus, and sodium in the diet can help to slow down the buildup of wastes.

Like other nephrologists, I attempt to control several major factors that can affect and help retard the progression of kidney disease. These major issues are blood pressure control, lowering of bad cholesterol, lowering and controlling blood-sugar levels, increasing physical activity, diet and weight reduction, and—last but not least—an adequate protein diet (not a high-protein diet). As part of weight reduction, I also emphasize salt restriction and the DASH diet.

With the advent and popularity of highly dangerous, unbalanced, and unhealthy forms of high-protein diets, such as the Atkins diet, a majority of these patients are at greater risk of worsening kidney function.

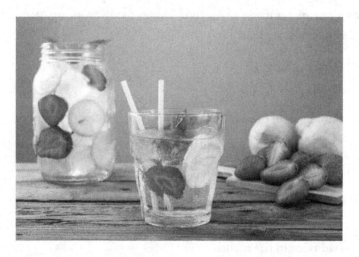

Water Is Essential for Detoxification

Given that 60 percent of your body weight is water, you need plenty of it to stay healthy. Furthermore, the fact that a large percentage of your body is water plays a significant role in all of your bodily functions and dysfunction.

All the biochemical reactions in your body occur in a water medium. Consequently, you cannot survive for more than a few days without water. On the other hand, you can live without food for a couple of months. Hence, to accomplish detoxification of your body, your total body water has to be replenished and cleaned. Simply put, you need water to detoxify your body!

Water vs. Other Beverages

There is a major difference between drinking water and other beverages. All beverages, including fruit juice cocktails, soft drinks, and coffee, may contain substances that are not healthy. In fact, some of these substances dehydrate your body. Caffeinated beverages act as diuretics and remove essential water from your body. Other beverages also contain dehydrating agents. Soft drinks contain phosphorus, sodium, and loads of sugars. These drinks may strain your body more than you think. They contain empty calories that you don't need. A can of regular cola, on average, contains two hundred empty and "bad" calories.

People with moderate to severe kidney disease, congestive heart failure, liver failure, or other conditions where there is serious body swelling should avoid drinking too much water and should consult their physicians. Nobody should ever undertake any type of diet without getting a doctor's approval of the dietary changes.

Furthermore, your kidneys have to work harder to remove the excess water from the body and that, too, must be taken into account. Drinking a couple of liters of water a day (eight glasses) has other benefits. Water can give you a sense of fullness and, to some extent, reduce the desire for food. Your body also has to burn a few calories to carry the weight of the fluid you drink. Your body will burn a few calories simply by carrying around the weight.

Taking all this into account, ingesting two liters of water per day results in a weight loss of about eight pounds of fat in a year!

Benefits of Water

+ Waste removal (getting rid of waste in stool, urine, and sweat)
+ Constipation relief
+ Body temperature regulation

- Asthma relief
- Kidney function improvement
- Joint lubrication (better mobility and hydration of the cartilage)
- Muscle function improvement
- Brain function (extremely sensitive to dehydration and overhydration)
- Migraine/headache reduction (in intensity and frequency)
- Pregnancy health (healthy fetus and amniotic fluid)
- Digestion efficiency (better bowel movements and metabolism)
- Metabolism improvement

Fiber for Detoxification

Insoluble fibers provide more volume and bulk to stool size and play a major role in reducing the risk for certain types of cancer. Insoluble fibers aid the passage of undigested material and waste through the bowel, preventing constipation and helping to rid the body of toxins. Unless your diet is high in fiber, you run the risk of getting constipated. Therefore, in addition to water, you need high fiber to eliminate toxins and waste and help the detoxification process.

Vitamins and Minerals as Antioxidants and their Natural Food Sources

Vitamin A Carotenoids

All colorful and brightly colored fruits and vegetables, carrots, squash, broccoli, sweet potatoes, tomatoes, kale, collards, cantaloupe, peaches, and apricots

All citrus fruits, all green leafy vegetables, green peppers, broccoli, strawberries, and tomatoes
Vitamin C
Vitamin E

Selenium

> All green leafy vegetables, nuts, seeds, whole grains, vegetable oil, and liver oil

> Fish, shellfish, meat, grains, eggs, poultry, and garlic

Substance	Food Sources
Flavonoids/quercetin	Shallots, beans, greens, apples
Ellagic acid	All berries, pomegranates
Indoles/isothiocyanates	Cabbage, radish, mustard, garlic
Terpenes/limonene	Citrus fruits
Polyphenols/catechin	Red grapes, tea, chocolate, cocoa

Detoxification Program

The main idea behind this detoxification program is to accomplish a safe and gentle cleansing and detoxification of your body. This program takes advantage of the three important components of a natural and gentle detoxification: water, fiber, and antioxidants.

This program is as follows:

Complete Version

> No alcohol throughout all the phases

> No caffeine or caffeinated beverages throughout all phases

> No meat, fish, poultry throughout all phases

> Phases can be as short as twenty-four hours to the maximum noted.

Phase 1

Day 1

Hydrate your body with water during the fasting period. Fast and don't eat anything in the next 8-12 hours if possible.

If you feel your blood-sugar level is dropping, you may drink fruit juices. Those allowed include pomegranate juice, orange juice, carrot juice, cranberry juice, and apple juice.

Day 2

Drink water and fruit juices with high-antioxidant properties: pomegranate, tomato, orange, cranberry, or carrot.

No solid food during this period, if possible.

Phase 2

Day 3

In the next twenty-four hours, drink more water. Make sure to take some multivitamins.

Start a diet of fruits, vegetables, and herbs, as much as you like.

Phase 3

Day 4

Even though other detox diets encourage you to undergo colonic irrigation to clean out your colon, I do not recommend this. The Antiox-Detox Soup recipe (page 00) can accomplish a gentle colonic irrigation and cleansing.

Eat the Antiox-Detox Soup for one day with lots of water intake. You have to make sure that you drink plenty of water or juices. This soup mixture will provide a large dose of antioxidants, fiber, and natural laxatives.

Day 5

Phase 4

During the fourth phase of detoxification, it is preferred that you eat fresh yogurt to introduce a healthy culture into your intestines. If you feel very hungry, you may start the L.O.V.E. diet program, or resume it if you are already on it.

Chew your food thoroughly, and drink at least ten to twelve glasses of water or carbonated water.

NOTE: *This detoxification method should only be used on a temporary basis, to be followed by a well-balanced and nutritious lifestyle approach.*

A Shorter Version

This program is a modification of the original plan.

No alcohol, caffeine, or caffeinated beverages should be consumed throughout all the phases. In addition, heavy meals such as meat, and fish, poultry should be avoided throughout all phases.

Day 1

Phase 1

In this phase, you should attempt to hydrate your cells and body as a whole with water for at least twenty-four hours. You should fast and not eat anything during the hydrating period, if possible. If you feel your blood-sugar level is dropping, you may drink fruit juices or have small snacks like fruits or vegetables. Allowed fruit juices: pomegranate juice, orange juice, carrot juice, cranberry juice, and apple juice.

Phase 2

Day 2

In the next twenty-four hours, drink more water. Make sure to take some multivitamins. Start a diet of fruits, vegetables, and herbs, as much as you like.

Phase 3

Day 3

Prepare the Antiox-Detox Soup, and eat it for the next twenty-four hours. Make sure to drink plenty of water or fruit juices. This soup mixture will provide a large dose of antioxidants, fiber, and natural laxatives.

Day 4

Phase 4

During the fourth phase of detoxification, it is preferred that you eat fresh yogurt to introduce a healthy culture into your intestines. If you feel very hungry, you may start the L.O.V.E. diet program or resume it if you are already on it.

Gentle Colonic Cleansing

I have developed a simple, one-phase, gentle colon-cleansing protocol using herbs, vegetables, and certain fruits. This simple detoxification method can be performed every other week instead of the more rigorous detox protocol detailed above. In this simple colon-cleansing protocol, a full day of eating this soup will cleanse your system. Of course, good hydration needs to be incorporated while colon cleansing in progress.

The ingredients of this Antiox-Detox Soup is any combination of the following vegetables. Of course, the more ingredients, the better the result!

Ingredients of Antiox-Detox Soup

Artichoke
Beets
Cabbage-green
Cabbage-red
Carrots
Celery
Chives
Fennel
Fennel Seed
Ginger
Leeks
Onions
Parsley
Pepper, red

Pepper, yellow
Prunes
Rhubarb
Scallion
Spinach
Tamarind
Turmeric
Turnip

Colonic Irrigation/Colon Hydrotherapy: Avoid These Dangerous Procedures

There are three types of colonic irrigation or colon hydrotherapy: (1) ordinary enema, (2) colonic irrigation, and (3) high colonic. The goal of this procedure is to flush built-up toxins from the bowel. A myth!

Colonic irrigation is very similar to an ordinary rectal enema but involves a larger quantity of liquid—usually a gallon. This liquid is pumped, with the use of gravity and a machine, into the large intestine via a tube placed high in the rectum. Colonic irrigation is an effort to wash and remove the contents of the colon.

A high colonic is a form of colonic irrigation in which an even larger quantity of liquid is used—twenty or more gallons. The types of liquids used in colonics may include soapsuds, coffee, coffee grounds, herbs, wheat grass extract, or many others that can be potentially irritating (373–377) It is believed—but yet to be proven—that these procedures detoxify the body and that regular "cleansing" is necessary to maintain one's health. Advocates of colonics have prescribed these procedures for many different ailments, including asthma, arthritis, chronic fatigue, and constipation. But proponents and advocates of colonics cannot refer to any clinical research showing any benefits.

It is theorized that undigested cellulose and bacteria can accumulate in the pockets and folds of the colon and back up the colon. Over time, elimination becomes increasingly difficult. As the feces builds up and becomes stagnant—it is theorized—it produces toxic substances. Furthermore, the body—again they theorize—regards toxic molecules of undigested foods as foreign bodies and produces antibodies to fight them. In the process, the antibodies can also destroy healthy tissue.

But the high colonics are not without risks and have sometimes been fatal (373–377). The risks associated with colonics include infection from contaminated equipment, rupture of the colon, and harmful disruption of the delicate chemical balance of the colon. The colon is the major site in the intestine that absorbs several electrolytes and minerals plus water to avoid loss in the feces. Thereby, colonics could cause some mineral and electrolyte deficiencies and disturbances of fluid balance of the body.

Like many other baseless fads and through vigorous Internet promotion, colonics are growing increasingly popular. Since there is no real evidence to support the health benefits of these practices, plus the fact that they could be dangerous, many doctors are concerned and discourage their practice.

Avoid Smoking

Proper nutrition goes beyond just eating the right food. There are other substances that have the capacity to harm your body and are detrimental to your overall health. In particular, smoking (nicotine) is harmful in many ways. There are numerous scientific studies demonstrating the ill effects of smoking on your body (378–380). Smoking can affect your heart, brain, kidneys, blood vessels, bladder, and lungs. Smoking also increases your risk of developing cancers of the mouth, throat, larynx, cervix, pancreas, esophagus, colon, rectum, kidney, and bladder.

Tobacco smoke is made up of thousands of compounds. These are a group of carcinogens and toxins that can damage your body and several important organs in your body. Among the toxins in cigarette smoke are glycerol, glycol, aldehydes, aromatic hydrocarbons, phenols, and poisonous gases of hydrogen cyanide and nitrogen oxide, as well as carbon monoxide.

There are approximately six hundred additives used in the manufacturing of cigarettes. The main components of tobacco smoke are nicotine, tar, and carbon monoxide. Nicotine is a powerful carcinogen and a strong mood-altering substance that reaches the brain quickly when you smoke a cigarette. In addition, nicotine is also extremely toxic. A moderate dose of thirty milligrams can be lethal. Tar is a combination of hundreds of chemicals, including toxins and carcinogens. Again, cardiovascular and circulatory disease, lung, bladder, and other cancers, and emphysema and chronic bronchitis have been linked to some of these substances.

Major Constituents of Tobacco Smoke

1-Methylpyrrolidine	2-, 3- and 4-Methylpyridines
2,5-dimethylpyrazine	2-Nitropropane
Acetaldehyde	Acetone
Acrolein	Acrylonitrile
Ammonia	Benzene
Benzo[a]pyrene	Bicyclohexyl
Crotonaldehyde	Cyclohexane
Cyclopentane	Dimethylamine
Ethylamine	Formaldehyde
Furfural	Hydrazine
Hydrogen cyanide	Methyl acrylate
Methyl chloride	Methylamine
Methylpyrazines and	Nicotine
Nitric oxide	Nitrogen dioxide
N-Nitrosamines	PAH
Propionaldehyde	Pyridine
Pyrrolidine	Tar
Trimethylamine	Urethane
Vinyl chloride	

Avoid Excessive Alcohol

Consumption of alcohol in moderate amounts may be good for you. Some epidemiological studies indicate that moderate drinkers (drinking one glass of wine per day) live longer than nondrinkers and heavy drinkers (359–370). The reasons are not clear. This benefit could be due to a number of lifestyle factors. Alcohol is a compound that can be rapidly absorbed from your gut and, hence, affect or alter your mood. Alcohol is a depressant, which can worsen depression. But, drinking alcohol can also make you feel relaxed, happy, and even euphoric. It can also affect you brain and decrease your physical coordination and mental judgment, leading to loss of inhibitions.

Alcohol intake in moderation is thought to be beneficial in reducing the risk of coronary disease. Indeed, it should be enjoyed in combination with high intakes of fruit and vegetables. This is the crux of the so-called "French paradox." Even though the French diet is high in fat, the death rate from cardiovascular disease remains relatively low. This cardiovascular benefit is thought to be due to consumption of red wine by the French.

Even though moderate drinking may have some benefits, it also carries increased health risks. Drinking too much causes serious problems. Frequency seems to be the key. Consuming smaller amounts several times a week, or one or two drinks daily or every other day, is most beneficial for your cardiovascular health. It seems that low, regular alcohol intake helps raise levels of HDL in your blood.

Alcohol lacks nutritional value and adds unneeded calories to your diet, which can contribute to weight gain and obesity.

How Much to Drink in a Day?

According to the US Department of Agriculture and Department of Health and Human Services, moderate drinking is described as follows:

- No more than one drink a day if you are a woman
- No more than one drink a day if you are over 60
- No more than two drinks a day if you are a man

One Drink = 5 ounces of wine, 12 ounces of beer, or 1.5 ounces of alcohol (381)

A daily rather than weekly amount is preferred. You should avoid drinking if you are pregnant or trying to conceive, taking medication, a recovering alcoholic, or under legal age. If you are not drinking, don't be encouraged to start drinking. There are other nutrients and food that offer the same benefits (red grape juice, pomegranate juice, and chocolate).

Benefits of Moderate Alcohol Consumption

+ Reduces your risk of developing heart disease
+ Reduces peripheral vascular disease
+ Reduces intermittent claudication (painful leg cramping)
+ Reduces risk of dying of a heart attack
+ Reduces your risk of strokes (ischemic strokes)
+ Reduces your risk of diabetes (controversial)

Risks of Excessive Alcohol Consumption

+ Increased cancers of gastrointestinal tract (oral, pharynx, larynx, esophageal, and liver)
+ Increased breast cancer in women
+ Increased risk of chronic pancreatitis
+ Increased levels of triglycerides (bad cholesterol) in the blood
+ Increased blood pressure
+ Increased risk of heart failure
+ Increased risk of stroke
+ Increased risk of cirrhosis of the liver
+ Increased depression and risk of suicide

It is important to note that all alcoholic drinks and cocktails are loaded with calories. Hence, if you intend to drink any type of alcoholic beverage, you need to factor it into your calorie count.

Caloric Content of Common Alcoholic Drinks

Drink	Caloric Content
Serving size approximately 250 ml	
Beer	100
Mild bitter, draught	70
Brown ale	80
Pale ale	90
Strong ale	200
Lager	90
Serving size approximately 125 ml	
Red wine	85
Sweet white wine	120
Dry white wine	85
Medium white wine	95
Sparkling white wine	95
Port	80
Sherry, dry	60

Chapter Ten

Pointers on Burning Calories

Use these tricks to eat less, eat healthier, burn more calories, and take in fewer calories.

Never skip a meal.

Don't stuff yourself. Stop eating before you feel full but are satiated.

Smell the aroma of food and spices.

Eat more salads.

Eat a good-sized salad before the main course. Eat as much as you can to fill your stomach. Make sure you have lots of variety in the salad mix. The more colorful the salad, the healthier it is. Remember, avoid processed salad dressing, and use more of the good oils, such as olive oil and grapeseed oil, in combination with lemon juice or vinegar.

Later, when the main course arrives, all you will do is just pick at it. This is a good weight-management strategy. Research shows that you can cut your intake by an average of one hundred calories when you start your meal with a large salad. The larger the salad, the more reduction in calorie intake you can achieve. Of course, salads must be low-calorie to help you manage your weight. To benefit from this "filling-up" effect of the pre-meal salad, you have to wait ten to twenty minutes before eating your main course.

Sit down every time you want to eat. Concentrate on what you are eating.

Chew your food more. Chew each bite at least ten to twenty times. This will allow you to fool your brain into thinking you have eaten a lot and allow you to taste the food and burn more calories.

Eat your food slowly. Don't rush, and don't wolf down the food! If you eat hurriedly, you might still eat the same amount after a large salad. Your body may not have enough time to sense its fullness.

Put smaller portions on your plate. In a study, it was shown that people usually eat more just because there is more food on the plate. The researchers reported that a person's amount of intake is governed by how much food is on his or her plate, not his or her appetite (382–399).

Drink more fluids with your meals.

Breathe deep and try to relax. Breathe better, and deeper! When you breathe more naturally and efficiently, it can influence your metabolism greatly and give you an overall sense of well-being.

Sing and dance anytime you can.

Eat more solid food. Since solid food requires chewing, it fools your brain. In addition, solid food stays longer in the stomach, since it requires more digestion. Therefore, the satiety and fullness sensation lasts longer. Remember: an apple is better than a glass of apple juice. Hence, avoid juices, shakes, and smoothies, if possible.

Eat more vegetables and fruits.

Hug as much as you can.

Take the stairs.

Eliminate bad calories. Eat fewer calories.

Eat more complex carbohydrates and whole grains.

Eat fewer fats.

Eat more foods that are high in vitamins A, C, E, B.

Drink more water.

Limit coffee and soft drinks.

Eliminate sugar, refined foods, preserved foods, and fat-laden snack foods.

Park at the end of the lot, and walk more.

Prepare the food yourself. Cook the food, and use more fresh ingredients. Avoid fast foods, frozen meals, and high-calorie snacks loaded with calories.

Some Pointers on Eating Out

Always start the meal with a large salad. Ask for salad dressing on the side, and use the salad dressings sparingly. Olive oil and vinegar salad dressings are preferable. Order smaller portion dishes and make sure to choose meals that are steamed, broiled, baked, roasted, poached, or stir-fried. Ask for your meal to be served without gravy and fat-containing sauces. It is a good idea to share the main course and especially the dessert. Choose desserts that are healthy and have fewer calories. Don't be afraid to take a portion of the food home with you.

Eat only when you're hungry.

Stop eating before you are full (but satiated), and leave a little bit of food on your plate.

Eat only when you are sitting and relaxed.

Pay attention to what you are eating, and do not be distracted.

Eat slowly.

If you are not enjoying the food, don't eat it.

Chapter Eleven

Take Care of Your Skin by Eating Well

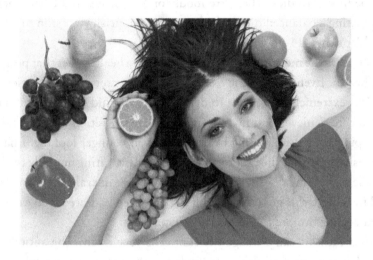

Healthy Skin and Its Importance to General Health

It is very important to realize that the skin is very important to your health. The skin—the epidermis—is not just a covering for your body. It is actually the largest organ in your body! Skin plays a vital role in maintaining health and fighting diseases. In addition, your skin releases toxins and wastes from your body through sweat glands, hence acting as a detoxification system.

The composition of sweat can vary among people and is influenced by many factors, such as emotional state, diet, and exercise. This explains why you may notice an oniony or garlicky odor on your skin after consuming a large amount of these foods.

Simply put, the composition of your sweat is almost similar to that of your plasma, except that sweat does not contain proteins. Therefore, sweat is like a filtrate of plasma that contains electrolytes like potassium, sodium, and chloride, and metabolic wastes like blood urea and lactic acid.

Furthermore, any water-soluble chemicals, like some drugs and metal ions, can also be excreted in sweat (400–413).

To acquire glowing, vibrant, and, younger-looking skin, you have to eat more of the healthy foods. The healthier the foods that you consume, the healthier and younger your skin will look. The reverse is also true. The less healthy foods you eat, the less vibrant your skin becomes. This can be seen as older-looking skin, sallow skin, dry skin, and more wrinkled skin, not to mention skin breakouts and conditions like eczema and acne, which may be linked to diet. There are foods for a healthier and better-looking skin. Eating a balanced diet is the best way to nourish your skin to attain a healthier skin (414–426).

Water is the most important component of a healthy diet that promotes skin health. Even though the exact amount of water required varies each day, it is extremely important to drink plenty of fluid (about eight glasses of water) to achieve good hydration. Adequate hydration plays a vital role in keeping your skin looking healthy and even younger looking. I have to emphasize here that the best form of liquid for hydrating not only the body but also your skin is clean, pure water. However, mineral water can also be used to achieve this goal. As a result of being well hydrated, you can sweat better and clear more toxins via the perspiration.

Free radicals can damage the skin cells very easily. The antioxidants and other phytochemicals in certain fruits and vegetables can protect the skin cells from damage. As a result, you protect your skin from premature aging. In this respect, fruits and vegetables may help keep your skin looking younger longer.

Healthy oils, as discussed in earlier chapters, are part of a well-balanced diet. Eating good-quality oils helps keep your skin lubricated and looking and feeling healthier overall. In addition, these oils contain essential fatty acids, which are important nutrients responsible for healthy skin cells. The best-known essential fatty acids are omega 3 and omega 6, which must be in balance for good health and better skin. For example, essential fatty acids can help the skin cells to hold the moisture better. As a result, your skin looks younger and plumper (414–420).

Another compound—polyphenols, mostly found in green tea—has also been studied for its effect on skin cells. A study published in the *Archives of Dermatology* showed that whether taken orally or applied to the skin, green tea reduced the risk of damage from ultraviolet light, such as the burning rays of the sun, and thus reduce the risk of skin cancer (428–431). Green tea also has anti-inflammatory properties that may also be beneficial to overall skin health (414, 417).

Selenium content of certain foods is paramount for healthy skin. Based on many studies, selenium plays a key role in not only the health of skin cells but also prevents damaged skin to worsen or progress to skin cancer and aging (428–450). Although selenium salts are toxic if ingested in large amounts, trace amounts of this element are not only necessary but vital for cellular functions. Selenium forms the active part of the very important class of enzymes needed to eliminate oxidative products that can accumulate and damage the cells in the body. These enzymes—glutathionperoxides and thioredoxin reductase—indirectly reduce and neutralize oxidized molecules in animals and even in some plants. In addition, selenium is also necessary for three known deiodinase enzymes that convert one thyroid hormone to another. In two clinical trials published in 2003 in the *British Journal of Dermatology* and the journal *Clinical and Experimental Dermatology*, it was shown that when levels of selenium were high, skin cells were less likely to suffer the kind of oxidative damage that can increase the risk of cancer. Another study found that oral doses of selenium, along with copper, vitamin E, and vitamin A, could prevent sunburn in human skin (428–467).

In addition to promoting better and healthier-looking skin by proper diet, you can improve the skin by applying certain natural products that can increase exfoliation of your skin as well as hydrate it. Furthermore, as mentioned previously, certain chemicals can promote skin health whether applied externally or consumed.

Alpha Hydroxy

Alpha hydroxy acid is a low molecular weight organic acid. Organic acids are thousands of degrees milder than mineral acids and are commonly found in fruits and fermented foods. Acetic acid, for example, is the organic acid that gives vinegar its characteristic sour taste.

Nowadays, alpha hydroxy acids are used extensively in cosmetics and dermatology clinics. They can either be used in lower concentration for daily use and gentle exfoliation or at higher concentration as a peeling agent. Furthermore, dermatologists and plastic surgeons use glycolic acid, an alpha hydroxy, to eliminate scarring, and decrease skin pigmentation and skin irregularities. How well these agents work depends on the number of peeling sessions and the contact time. Dermatologists and plastic surgeons are using these compounds as an effective anti-aging ingredient to combat the loss of skin elasticity and wrinkling associated with aging.

Fruits Are a Major Source of Alpha Hydroxy

Alpha hydroxy acids—also known as fruit acids—are chemicals found in all kinds of fruits. Actually, they are also isolated from fruits and sold commercially. Alpha hydroxy acids can be isolated from fermentation of natural products.

It is well known that many cultures have used the power of alpha hydroxy by using facial masks made from yogurt, honey, and fruits. For example, Egyptian queens took baths in sour milk to improve their skin condition.

Major Sources of Alpha Hydroxy

Malic acid is found in apples.
Citric acid is found in all citrus fruits.
Glycolic acid is found in honey and sugarcane.
Lactic acid is found in sour milk.
Tartaric acid is found in wine.

One of the most common alpha hydroxy acids in use is glycolic acid, because it is presumed to penetrate skin easier. Lactic acid, on the other hand, has a larger molecular size than glycolic acid. Some people mistakenly characterize salicylic acid or retinoic acid as an alpha hydroxy acid.

Alpha hydroxy acids act as a hydrating agent by moisturizing the outer layer of the epidermis and, as a result, make the skin softer and more flexible. They also act as an exfoliant, getting rid of the dead cells that form at the surface of the skin.

The efficacy of an alpha hydroxy acid when used as an exfoliating agent depends on the concentration of the acid and the pH of the medium in which it is used. But surprisingly, it does not depend on the specific alpha hydroxy acid used.

Make Your Own Anti-Aging Cream!

Wine Yogurt Honey Apple Sugarcane
Oat bran (ground)
Green tea (leaf)

This alpha hydroxy acid lotion should give you less dramatic results than retin-A, but it is also less likely to irritate your skin. However, over time you get the same benefits.

To neutralize the harmful effects of the oxidants and the free radicals on your body, it is essential to include large doses of natural antioxidants in your diet. These antioxidants include antioxidant-rich foods, such as avocado, colorful sweet peppers, all kinds of berries, melons, all green leafy vegetables, all citrus fruits, squash, tomatoes, and pineapples. You can also get a good supply of antioxidants from herbs and spices, such as dill, coriander, rosemary, sage, thyme, mint, fennel, garlic, and ginger. It is also important to have a diet with adequate protein.

Chapter Twelve

The Plateau Principle in Diet
and the Science of Muscle and Body Confusion

The Plateau Principle

Professor Wilbur Olin Atwater, an American chemist known for his studies of human nutrition and metabolism, developed the first database of food composition in the United States. Atwater is best known for his studies of human nutrition. He studied respiration and metabolism in animals and in humans. In order to study these topics, he invented and utilized a machine called the respiration calorimeter. The calorimeter aided studies in food analysis, dietary evolution, work energy consumption, and digestible foods. In addition, it measured the human metabolism balance by analyzing the heat produced and metabolic rate by a person performing certain physical activities.

Dr. Atwater recognized that the response to excessive or insufficient nutrient and calorie intake resulted in an adjustment by the body to increase its efficiency in metabolism that would result in a plateau.

Dr. Atwater wrote about his observations from the findings of numerous experiments that "when the nutrients are fed in large excess, the body may continue for a time to store away part of the extra material, but after it has accumulated a certain amount, it refuses to take on more, and the daily consumption equals the supply even when this involves great waste" (605). Astonishingly, the plateau principle exists not only in weight-loss programs but also in other fields, such as biochemistry, physiology, and nutrition (606–612).

Plateaus During Dieting and Weight-Loss Period

The weight-loss plateau follows a typical pattern. During the initial few weeks of losing weight, a rapid drop in body weight is normal. This weight loss is due to reduced intake of food and ultimately calories. As a result, your body attempts to provide the needed calories by releasing stores of glycogen (a highly compacted form of carbohydrate) stored in the muscles and liver. As a consequence of burning glycogen for calories, water is generated. Interestingly, for every ounce of burning glycogen, four ounces of water is generated resulting in substantial weight loss that is mostly water!

Therefore, it is especially common for all people who are trying to lose weight to experience plateaus after several weeks of successful weight reduction. The principle of the weight-loss plateau has been studied in calorie-restriction experiments, which has shed light on the mechanism of this annoying phenomenon (613).

Caloric Restriction

Caloric restriction is a stringent dietary routine that has been shown to have health benefits in studies on many animals, including mice, primates, and worms (614–616). In the caloric-restriction experiments, the mice are kept on a diet that is healthy but has about 30 percent fewer calories than a normal diet. Interestingly, the mice live 30 or 40 percent longer than usual, with the only side effect of being less fertile. In addition, this diet appears to protect mice from degenerative disease, which may explain the increased longevity.

It is self-evident that humans cannot follow and maintain such a restricted diet. People find it almost impossible to maintain such a drastic caloric restriction (30 percent drop in caloric requirement). As a result, caloric restriction as a recipe for increased longevity has remained a scientific curiosity for many decades. Therefore, there is a great race among scientists to develop a medicine that would "trick" the body into thinking it is on a caloric-restriction diet (617–619).

A discovery of single genes that function primarily in regulation of growth has achieved a statistically significant increase in life span in animal experiments (614, 620–622). This single gene seems to act through the same biochemical pathways through which the caloric-restriction diet increases longevity.

Dangers of Severe Caloric Restriction

The Minnesota Starvation (semi-starvation) Experiment was a clinical study performed by Ancel Keys et al. at the University of Minnesota between 1944 and 1945 (623, 624). The investigation was designed to determine the physiological and psychological effects of severe and prolonged caloric and dietary restriction and the effectiveness of dietary-rehabilitation strategies.

The study was divided into three phases: a twelve-week control phase; a twenty-four-week starvation phase, over which the caloric restriction caused each participants to lose approximately 25 percent of their pre-starvation body weight; and a recovery phase, where various rehabilitative diets were used to nourish the volunteers back to baseline. The results were published in 1950 (623–625).

Data from the Minnesota Starvation Experiment demonstrate that during food restriction, total body mass, fat mass, and lean body mass follow an exponential approach to a new steady-state. The observation that body mass changes exponentially during partial or complete starvation seems to be a general feature of adaptation to energy restriction.

There were other findings that were very interesting though disturbing. For example, prolonged semi-starvation produced significant increases in depression, hysteria, and hypochondriasis. There were extreme reactions to the psychological effects during the experiment, including self-mutilation. Study subjects exhibited a preoccupation with food, both during the starvation period and the rehabilitation phase. Sexual interest was drastically reduced, and the subjects showed signs of social withdrawal and isolation. Additionally, the subjects reported a decline in concentration, comprehension, and judgment capabilities. Astonishingly, the study subjects showed marked declines in physiological processes indicative of decreases in each subject's basal metabolic rate, which reflected in their body temperature, respiration, and heart-rate reduction (623–624).

The fact that weight loss reduces the metabolic rate is supported by clinical research. In a study by Chaput et al., heat production was reduced by 30 percent in obese men after a weight-loss program, and this led to resistance to further lose body weight (626). Furthermore, maintenance of a body weight at a level 10 percent or more below the initial weight was associated with a lower reduction in total energy expenditure in the subjects who had never been obese compared to the obese subjects. In addition, resting energy expenditure and nonresting energy expenditure decreased in both groups of subjects. Maintenance of body weight at a level 10 percent above the usual weight was associated with an increase in total energy expenditure, which was greater in the subjects who had never been obese compared to the obese subjects. Whether body mass increases or decreases, there are adjustments in resting energy expenditure (BMR), and nonresting energy expenditures all oppose further change. Maintenance of a reduced or elevated body weight is associated with compensatory changes in energy expenditure. This change in energy expenditure and metabolism opposes the maintenance of a body weight that is different from the usual weight. These compensatory changes in metabolism may account for the poor long-term efficacy of many weight-loss programs and diets (626–627).

It is an inevitable truth that almost everyone reaches a weight-loss plateau at some point in their diet. The reason underlying this physiological plateau is that the human body is extremely efficient and can adapt to many different extreme situations, including calorie restriction. The ultimate objective of the body is to keep energy intake and output in balance.

A weight-loss plateau occurs because your metabolism slows as you lose weight and your body becomes more efficient. When you lose weight, you lose both fat and lean tissue. It is generally not true that overweight people have a slower metabolism. But it is true that the higher your weight, the higher your body's metabolic rate. Your weight-loss efforts result in a new body weight and a new equilibrium, with your body metabolism slowing down proportionately.

It should be emphasized that the energy generated from food intake is expended largely to fight against gravity. Therefore, as you lose weight, the amount of calories that you need to burn throughout the day to fight against gravity lessens in addition to the effectiveness of a given workout. Furthermore, with exercise, your body and muscles gain greater efficiency, which is reflected in your workout: you don't get tired or run out of breath as easily as when you started the exercise regimen.

As a consequence of these factors, no matter how much you exercise and lower your calorie and food intake, you can barely break through this plateau. Ultimately, most of your efforts to lose weight are spent in maintaining that weigh plateau. This can be very disappointing and counterproductive. In fact, people give up on their diet or new way of life, since it seems to them that they have reached an insurmountable point in their weight loss. The only way to get past this plateau is to increase your metabolism by decreasing calorie intake, increasing activity level, and confusing your muscles!

Muscle Confusion Technique

Anyone who has trained for a sport or for weight loss has more than likely experienced plateaus, and this has given rise to various strategies to continue improving this dreadful point in any form of diet or weight-loss program (628). In order to overcome this phenomenon, you must change your physical activities and exercise routines to achieve the concept of muscle confusion.

Since physical activity is a major component of the weight-loss and weight-management program, it is inevitable that you will reach a plateau at some point in your progress. A few short weeks after starting your diet, your body—the ultimate machine—can get used to the type of exercises and physical activities that you are performing. In addition, your metabolism gets adjusted to the new calorie intake. So, as part of the L.O.V.E. diet program, you need to plan for and be ready to tackle this major issue and to avoid it if possible.

The best way to avoid or break through this plateau effect is to change your physical activities daily. By doing so, you confuse your body, and ultimately your muscles, and prevent them from becoming too efficient at one particular exercise or group of muscle activities.

Perform physical activities that are different from one another to ensure that you rotate through different groups of muscles. This rotation will also allow one muscle group to rest while you are using a different group of muscles. It is during the rest phase that you start to build and develop your muscles. Furthermore, other components of your body (tendons, ligaments, and joints) will be exercised evenly rather than repeatedly, thus avoiding any undue injuries. This resting/healing phase can be achieved even by changing the length of time and or the level of the activities you are performing daily (e.g., one hour vs. half an hour of exercise or walking vs. brisk walking or jogging).

Body/muscle confusion can be achieved very easily. Your body does not know what equipment you are using to achieve your weight loss. All the body understands is that you are training or using certain groups of muscles on daily basis. For example, if you play tennis ever day, your body becomes very efficient and conditioned for that particular sport. However, if you start weight lifting, since you have not exercised other groups of muscles involved in weight lifting, you will feel the effects of this strenuous exercise. Not all sports or physical activities use the same group(s) of muscles. So, by changing your physical activities and exercise daily, you will achieve the goal of optimizing all your muscle and avoiding or minimizing the plateau effect.

Ways to Break Through the Weight-Loss Plateau

1. Exercise with more intensity or exercise harder.

2. Change your exercise routine daily, if not weekly. Do a different exercise every day or at most every week.

3. Exercise in a colder environment if possible.

4. Swim in a colder pool of water.

5. Calorie cycling. Calorie cycling is the process of varying daily calorie intake while maintaining the same weekly intake. For example, instead of consuming your precise required calorie requirements, you can alter the amount on different days, but make sure the total calorie per week remains the same.

6. Strength training. Make sure you work out your muscles as part of your routine exercise.

7. Change meal frequency. Cycle your calories.

8. Tighten up your diet.

9. Increase your meal frequency while keeping the calories within goal.

10. Change duration of your exercise.

11. Change how often you exercise.

12. Change the intensity of your workouts.

13. Track your progress throughout your training.

14. Drink plenty of water (cold water is even better).

Chapter Thirteen

The Professor's Concluding Thoughts

As I have mentioned before, it is vital and extremely important that you approach any goal you set for yourself as a mind-body-spirit experience. After all, you are a combination of these three, interconnected, interdependent, and inseparable components. It is impossible to concentrate on one component and let go of the others.

So, go ahead and take care of the physical body by giving attention to your mind and your soul. If these components are connected, you as an individual will be at peace and in balance.

I hope that by reading this book you have realized the full potential of this healthy and nutritious diet—or as I like to say, a pathway to a healthier you. I am sure that you have realized that this "diet" is a holistic approach to nourishing your body and your soul. This is one of the aspects of this diet that makes it stand apart from all other diet programs and fad diets.

Remember, you have the power to become a healthier you and, as a consequence, become more youthful. But to achieve this goal, you have to start now; don't delay until tomorrow. Many people make the mistake of saying, "I will start my diet tomorrow," while they gorge on unhealthy calories devoid of nutritious food. Remember that every day you start this multifaceted approach to diet and a new way of life, you are closer to better living. If possible, incorporate it into your life by sharing it with your loved ones. You can stick to your diet if everyone in the family follows it! It would be very difficult to change the lifestyle, so introduce things one step at a time. As you do this, you will realize many of these lifestyle changes are interconnected. By learning about good, nutritious food and how to distinguish it from junk food, you will be able to change your diet in many positive ways. For example, by following your diet and eating more fruits, you will realize that you have accomplished several important goals at the same time: you ate more fiber, more unrefined food, more antioxidants, and

Mordechai S. Nosrati, MD

more vitamins and minerals! Amazingly, one simple act will have so many ramifications. And this is another important characteristic and benefit of the L.O.V.E. diet program. The food, your body, your mind, and your soul are all interconnected. One positive step has many other positive effects that reverberate in your life and your health status.

Make sure you set reasonable goals, and each time you achieve one, set another achievable goal. So, start your new way of life. Get up and move. Be more active, and eat healthfully. And last but not least, get in touch with your mind and soul, and embrace spirituality to make you not only healthier but a well-balanced and complete being.

228

Endnotes

1.   Projecting the Number of Patients with End-Stage Renal Disease in the United States to the Year 2015 J Am Soc Nephrol 16: 3736–3741, 2005.

2.   http://www.kidneyfund.org/AboutAKF/Newsroom_020425.htm.

3.   http://www.kidney.org/professionals/kdoqi/guideline_diabetes/guide5. htm.

4.   Meyer, TW, Anderson, SA, Rennke, HG, Brenner, BM. Reversing glomerular hypertension stabilizes established glomerular injury. Kidney Int 1987; 31: 752.

5.   Zatz, R, Meyer, TW, Rennke, HG, Brenner, BM. Predominance of hemodynamic rather than etabolic factors in the pathogenesis of diabetic nephropathy. Proc Natl Acad Sci USA 1985; 82: 5963.

6.   Miller, PL, Scholey, JW, Rennke, HG, Meyer, TW. Glomerular hypertrophy aggravates epithelial cell injury in nephrotic rats. J Clin Invest 1990; 85: 1119.

7.   Fukui, M, Nakamura, T, Ebihara, I, et al. Low-protein diet attenuates increased gene expression of platelet-derived growth factor and transforming growth factor-ß in experimental glomerular sclerosis. J Lab Clin Med 1993; 121:224.

8.   Nakamura, T, Fukui, M, Ebihara, I, et al. Low protein diet blunts the rise in glomerular gene expression in focal glomerulosclerosis. Kidney Int 1994; 45: 1593.

9.   Woods, LL. Mechanisms of renal hemodynamic regulation in response to protein feeding. Kidney Int 1993; 44: 659.

10. King, AJ, Levey, AS. Dietary protein and renal function. J Am Soc Nephrol 1993; 3: 1723.

11. Nakamura, H, Ho, S, Ebe, N, Shibata, A. Renal effects of different types of proteins in healthy volunteers and diabetic patients. Diabetes Care 1993; 16: 1071.

12. http://www.who.int/dietphysicalactivity/publications/facts/obesity/en.

13. http://www.caloriecontrol.org/about-the-council.

14. http://www.cdc.gov/obesity/defining.html.

15. Nutrition and Kidney Disease: A New Era: Dietary Protein Intake and Kidney Disease in Western Diet; Pecoits-Filho R Suzuki. Contrib Nephrol. Basel, Karger, 2007, vol 155, pp 102–112.

16. Knight, EL. The Impact of Protein Intake on Renal Function Decline in Women with Normal Renal Function or Mild Renal Insufficiency: Annals of Internal Medicine 18 March 2003 | Volume 138 Issue 6 | Pages 460–467

17. Effect of Low-Carbohydrate High-Protein Diets on Acid-Base Balance, Stone-Forming Propensity, and Calcium Metabolism. American Journal of Kidney Diseases 40(2002):265.

18. Sharman, MJ, Kraemer, WJ, Love, DM, et al. A ketogenic diet favorably affects serum biomarkers for cardiovascular disease in normal-weight men. J Nutr 2002 Jul;132(7):1879–1885.

19. De Stefani, S, Fierro, EL, Mendilaharsu, M, et al. 1998. Meat intake, "mate" drinking and renal cell cancer in Uruguay: a case-control study. Br. J. Cancer 78 (9): 1239–43.

20. Risch, HAM, Jain, M, Marrett, LD, and Howe, GR. 1994. Dietary fat intake and risk of epithelial ovarian cancer. J. Nat. Cancer Inst. 86 (18): 1409–15.

21. Pillow, PC, Hursting, SD, Duphorne, CM, et al. 1997. Case-control assessment of diet and lung cancer risk in African Americans and Mexican Americans. Nutr. Cancer 29 (2):169–73

22. Alavania, MC, Brown, CC, Swanson, C, and Brownson, RC. 1993. Saturated fat intake and lung cancer risk amoung nonsmoking women in Missouri. J. Nat. Cancer Inst. 85(23): 1906–16.

23. Kelemen, LE, Kushi, LH, Jacobs DR, Jr., Cerhan, JR. Associations of Dietary Protein with Disease and Mortality in a Prospective Study of Postmenopausal Women. Am J Epidemiol 2005;161:239–249

24. http://www.atkinsdietalert.org/advisory.html

25. Coresh, J, Selvin, E, Stevens, LA, et al. Prevalence of chronic kidney disease in the United States. JAMA. 2007:298:2038–47.

26. Plantinga, LC, Boulware, LE, Coresh, J, et al. Patient awareness of chronic kidney disease: trends and predictors. Arch Intern Med.2008;168(20):2268–75.

27. A Low-Carbohydrate, Ketogenic Diet versus a Low-Fat Diet To Treat Obesity and Hyperlipidemia; A Randomized, Controlled Trial. Annals of Internal Medicine 140(2004):769.

28. Berkman, LF, and Glass, T. "Social Integration, Social Networks, Social Support, and Health," in Social Epidemiology, ed. L.F. Berkman and I. Kawachi (New York: Oxford University Press, 2000), 137–173.

29. Oscillations in "brain–body–mind"—A holistic view including the autonomous system. Brain Research, Volume 1235, 15 October 2008, Pages 2–11

30. Vanderwolf, CH. Brain, Behavior, and Mind: What do we know and What can we Know? Neuroscience & Biobehavioral Reviews, Volume 22, Issue 2, March 1998, Pages 125–142.

31. May Loo, M. Mind/Body Approaches: Biofeedback, Hypnosis, Spirituality; Integrative Medicine for Children (First Edition), 2009, Pages 5–14.

32. Love and Survival, the Scientific Basis for the Healing Power of Intimacy (HarperCollins, 1998).

33. Reis, H. co-editor, Encyclopedia of Human Relationships. Department of Health and Human Services: "The Effects of Marriage on Health: A Synthesis of Recent Research Evidence."

34. WebMD Health News "Happy Marriage, Better Blood Pressure." Arthur Aron, PhD, Annual meeting of the Society for Neuroscience, Washington, D.C., Nov. 15–19 2008.

35. WebMD Health News: "The Health Perks of Marriage." Psychological Science, December 2006.

36. Psychosomatic Medicine, November 2006.

37. Archives of General Psychiatry, December 2005.

38. WebMD Health News: "For Happiness, Seek Family, Not Fortune." (ref 8–14)

39. http://www.heartmath.org/research/science-of-the-heart-emotional-balance.html

40. Justice, B. "Who gets sick: how beliefs, moods, and thoughts affect your health" In cooperation with Peak Press; New York: Distributed by St. Martin's Press, c1988.

41. http://seniors-health-   medicare.suite101.com/article.cfm/health_benefits_of_pet_ownership_among_elderly

42. http://www.webmd.com/balance/features/spirituality-may-help-people-live-longer "People who attend religious services at least once a week are less likely to die in a given period of time than people who attend services less often."

43. Sachs-Ericsson, N. Religious Attendance Reduces Cognitive Decline Among Older Women with High Levels of Depressive Symptoms, J Gerontol A Biol Sci Med Sci (2009) 64A (12): 1283–1289.

44. Idler, EL, McLaughlin, J, Kasl, S. Religion and the Quality of Life in the Last Year of Life: J Gerontol B Psychol Sci Soc Sci (2009) 64B (4): 528–537.

45. Hill, TD. Religious Attendance and Mortality: An 8-Year Follow-Up of Older Mexican Americans: J Gerontol B Psychol Sci Soc Sci (2005) 60 (2): S102–S109.

46. http://www.modia.org/priere/jewish-meditation.html

47. Tart, C. "Adapting Eastern spiritual teachings to Western culture." The Journal of Transpersonal Psychology 22: 149–166.

48. Everly, GS, Lating, JM. A clinical guide to the treatment of human stress response. 2002 ISBN 0306466201 page 199.

49. Joseph, M. 1998, The effect of strong religious beliefs on coping with stress Stress Medicine. Vol 14(4), Oct 1998, 219–224.

50. Aftlansas, L, Golosheykin, S. Non-linear dynamic complexity of the human EEG during meditation. Journal Neurosci Lett. 2002 Sep 20;330(2):143–6.

51. Aftlansas, L, Golosheykin, S. Impact of regular meditation practice on EEG activity at rest and during evoked negative emotions. Journal Int J Neurosci. 2005 Jun;115(6):893–909.

52. Aftnas, LI, Golcheikeine, SA. Human anterior and frontal midline theta and lower alpha reflect emotionally positive state and internalized attention: high resolution EEG investigation of meditation. Journal Neuroscience Letters 310 (2001) 57–60.

53. Robertson, DS, Robertson, CP. "Snowbird Diet" Warner Books, ISBN 0-446-38283-3.

54. Science News: April 10th, 2010; Vol.177 #8/Feature Keeping Time:New findings show how circadian clocks make the body tick.

55. Hobson, JA. "Sleep and the Immune System" The Chemistry of Conscious States: How The Brain Changes Its Mind. 1994.

56. Blakeslee, S. Mystery of Sleep Yields as Studies Reveal Immune Tie. The New York Times: Thursday, October 8, 2009.

57. Creativity and problem solving are directly linked to adequate sleep. (Nature, Jan. 21, 2004)

58. Poor sleep linked to obesity, other ills; Associated Press Wed., May 7, 2008.

59. http://health.dailynewscentral.com/content/view/2677.

60. Spiegel, K, Leproult, R, Van Cauter, E. Impact of sleep debt on metabolic and endocrine function. Lancet. 1999;354:1435–1439. Abstract.

61. Vgontzas, AN, Zoumakis, E, Boxler, EO, et al. Adverse effects of modest sleep restriction on sleepiness, performance, and inflammatory cytokines. J Clin Endocrinol Metab. 2004;89:2119–2126. Abstract

62. Spiegel, K, Tasali, E, Peney, P, et al. Sleep curtailment in healthy young men is associated with decreased leptin levels: elevated ghrelin levels and increased hunger and appetite. Ann Intern Med. 2004;141:846–850. Abstract

63. Leproult, R, Copinschi, G, Buxton, O, et al. Sleep loss results in an elevation of cortisol levels the next evening, Sleep. 1997;20:865–870.

64. Spiegel, K, Leproult, R, Colecchia, EF, et al. Adaptation of the 24-h growth hormone profile to a state of sleep debt. Am J Physiol Regul Integr Comp Physiol. 2000;279:R874–R883. Abstract

65. Van Oyen, C, Witvilet, TE, Ludwig, and Vander Lann, KL. "Granting Forgiveness or Harboring Grudges: Implications for Emotions, Physiology and Health," Psychological Science no. 12 (2001):117–23.

66. American Psychological Association. "Forgiveness: A Sampling of Research Results." 2006.

67. http://www.forgiveness-institute.org/html/process_model.htm.

68. Maltby, J, Wood, AM, Day, L, Kon, TWH, Colley, A, and Linley, PA. (2008). Personality predictors of levels of forgiveness two and a half years after the transgression. Journal of Research in Personality, 42, 1088–1094.

69. "Forgiving (Campaign for Forgiveness Research)." 2006.

70. Sarinopoulos, S. "Forgiveness and Physical Health: A Doctoral Dissertation Summary," World of Forgiveness no. 2 (2000): 16–18.

71. Luskin, F. Forgive for Good: A Proven Prescription for Health and Happiness (Harper, 2002).

72. Easterbrook, G. "Forgiveness is Good for Your Health." 2006.

73. Kleinsmith, LJ, et al. Paired-associate learning as a function of arousal and interpolated interval. J. Exp. Psych. 1963; 65: 190.

74. Bradley, MM, Greenwald, MK, Petry, MC, Lang, PJ. Remembering pictures: pleasure and arousal in memory. J. Exp. Psych. Learn. Mem Cognition. 1992; 18: 379.

75. Neisser, U, et al. Remembering the earthquake: direct experience vs. hearing the news. Memory. 1996; 4: 337.

76. Bohannon, JN. Flashbulb memories for the space shuttle disaster: a tale of two theories. Cognition. 1988; 2: 179.

77. Roozendaal, B, et al. Dose-dependent suppression of adreno-cortical activity with metyrapone: effects on emotion learning. Psychoneuroendocrinology. 1996; 21: 681.

78. Vazdarjanova, A, McGaugh, JL. Basolateral amygdala is not critical for cognitive memory of contextual fear conditioning. Proc. Nat. Acad. Sci. USA. 1998; 95: 15003.

79. de Kloet, ER, Oitzl, MS, Joëls, M. Stress and cognition: are glucocorticoids good or bad guys? Trends Neurosci. 1999; 22: 422.

80. McGaugh, JL. Memory: a century of consolidation. Science. 2000; 287: 248.

81. McGaugh, JL. The amygdala modulates the consolidation of memories of emotionally arousing experiences. Annu. Rev. Neurosci. 2004; 27: 1.

82. Roozendaal, B. Glucocorticoids and the regulation of memory consolidation. Psychoneuroendocrinology. 2000; 25: 213.

83. McIntyre, CK, Roozendaal, B. Frontiers in Neuroscience; Chapter 13: Adrenal Stress Hormones and Enhanced Memory for Emotionally Arousing Experiences.

84. van der Kolk, BA. The Dana Foundation: In Terror's Grip: Healing the Ravages of Trauma, January 1, 2002 http://www.obesity.org/statistics.

85. Wang, N, et al. Brain dopamine and obesity Lancet 2001; 357: 354–57

86. Martel, P, Fantino, M. Mesolimbic dopaminergic system activity as afunction of food reward: a microdialysis study. Pharmacol Biochem Behav 1996; 53: 221–26.

87. Baptista, T. Body weight gain induced by antipsychotic drugs:mechanisms and management. Acta Psychiatr Scand 1999; 100: 3–16.

88. Towell, A, Muscat, R, Willner, P. Behavioural microanalysis of the role of dopamine in amphetamine anorexia. Pharmacol Biochem Behav 1988; 30: 641–48.

89. http://www.newmaterials.com/Customisation/News/Nanotechnology/ Nanotechnology/Mere_sightsme ll_of_food_spikes_levels_of_brain_ pleasure_chemical.asp.

90. http://www.bnl.gov/medical/RCIBI/addiction.asp.

91. Physiological effects in aromatherapy; Tapanee HongratanaworakitSongklanakarin J. Sci. Technol. Vol. 26 No. 1 Jan.– Feb. 2004.

92. Lorig, TS, Schwartz, GE. 1988. Brain and odor I. Alteration of human EEG by odor administration. Psychobiology, 16: 281–289.

93. Lorig, TS. 1989. Human EEG and odor response. Progress in Neurobiology, 285, 1–11. In: Aroma- Chology: A status review (Ed. by Jellinek, J.S.), Cosmet. & Toiletr., 109: 83–101.

94. Manley, CH. 1993. Psychological effect of odor. Crit. Rev. Food Sci. Nutr., 33: 57–62.

95. Miyazaki, Y, Takeuchi, S, Yatagai, M, and Koboyashi, S. 1991. The effects of essential oils on mood in humans. Chem. Senses, 16: 1984.

96. Nagai, H, Nakamura, M, Fujii, W, Inui, T, and Askura, Y. 1991. Effects of odors on humans II: Reducing effects of mental stress and fatigue. Chem. Senses, 16: 198.

97. Nagakawa, M, Nagai, H, and Inui, T. 1992. Evaluation of drowsiness by EEGs-Odors controlling drowsiness. Fragrance J., 20 (10): 68–72.

98. Parasuraman, R, Warm, JS, and Dember, WN. 1992. Effects of olfactory stimulation on skin conductance and event-related brain potentials during visual induced attention, Progress Report no. 6 to Fragrance Research Fund.

99. Prokasy, WF, and Raskin, DC. 1973. Electrodermal activity in psychological research, Academic Press, New York.

100. Schwartz, MW, et al. 1988. Psychology, 15: 281; cited according reference of Manley, C. H. 1993. Psychological effect of odor. Crit. Rev. Food Sci. Nutr., 33(1): 57–62.

101. Sugano, H. 1988. Psychophysiological studies of fragrances. In Perfumery: The Psychology and Biology of Fragrance, Chapman & Hill: New York, pp. 221–228.

102. Sugano, H. 1989. Effects of odors on mental function. Chem. Senses, 14: 303. Tisserand, R. 1977. The Art of Aromatherapy. C.W. Daniel, Essex.

103. The Impact of Nonclinical Factors on Repeat Cesarean Section JAMA, Jan 1991; 265: 59–63.

104. Opinion Leaders vs Audit and Feedback to Implement Practice Guidelines: Delivery After Previous Cesarean Section JAMA, May 1991; 265: 2202–2207.

105. van der Kolk, BA. The Dana Foundation: In Terror's Grip: Healing the Ravages of Trauma, January 1, 2002 http://www.obesity.org/statistics.

106. Prieto, JM. Depression as Predictor of Mortality Among Cancer Patients After Stem-Cell Transplantation Journal of Clinical Oncology, Vol 23, No 25 (September 1), 2005: pp. 6063–6071.

107. Depression, Pain, and Aging Karp and Reynolds Focus.2009; 7: 17–27.

108. Lett, HS. Depression as a Risk Factor for Coronary Artery Disease: Evidence, Mechanisms, and Treatment Psychosomatic Medicine 66:305–315 (2004).

109. Roan, S. The mind's role comes into focus, Los Angeles Times January 20, 2003 (48–52).

110. Bennett, MP. The effect of mirthful laughter on stress and natural killer cell activity. Altern Ther Health Med. 2003 Mar–Apr; 9(2):38–45.

111. JNCI Journal of the National Cancer Institute 1995 87(5):342–343.

112. Doskoch, P. Happily ever laughter. Psychol Today. 1996;29(4):32.

113. Meyer, M. Laughter: It's good medicine. Better Homes Gardens. 1997;74(4):72–76.

114. Traynor, D. Laugh it off. Am Fitness. 1997;15(3):56–58.

115. Bakerman, H. Humor as a nursing intervention. Axon. 1997;18(3):56–61.

116. Fry, W. The physiologic effects of humor, mirth, and laughter. JAMA.1992;267(13):1857–1858.

117. Erdman, L. Laughter therapy for patients with cancer. Oncol Nurs Forum.1991;18(8):1359–1363.

118. Gilligan, B. A positive coping strategy: humor in the oncology setting. Prof Nurse.1993;8(4):231–233.

119. Rosenberg, L. A qualitative investigation of the use of humor by emergency personnel as a strategy for coping with stress. J Emerg Nurs. 1991;17:197–203.

120. Eyer, D. Mother–Infant Bonding: A Scientific Fiction (New Haven, Conn.: Yale University Press, 1992).

121. Suomi, SJ. "Touch and the Immune System in Rhesus Monkeys," in Field, Touch in Early Development, 89–103.

122. Field, TM, et al. "Tactile/Kinesthetic Stimulation Effects on Preterm Neonates," Pediatrics 77 (1986): 654–58.

123. Polan, HJ, and Ward, MJ. "Role of the Mother's Touch in Failure to Thrive: A Preliminary Investigation," Journal of the American Academy of Child and Adolescent Psychiatry 33, no. 8 (1994): 1098–1105.

124. Fishman, E, Turkheimer, E, and DeGood, DE. "Touch Relieves Stress and Pain," Journal of Behavioral Medicine 18, no. 1 (1995): 69–79.

125. Gupta, MA, and Schork, NJ. "Touch Deprivation Has an Adverse Effect on Body Image: Some Preliminary Observations," International Journal of Eating Disorders no. 2 (1995): 185–89.

126. Gupta, MA, et al. "Perceived Touch Deprivation and Body Image: Some Observations among Eating Disordered and Non-Clinical Subjects," Journal of Psychosomatic Research 39, no. 4 (1995): 459–64.

127. Traina, C. Touch on Trial: Power and the Right to Physical Affection. Journal of the Society of Christian Ethics, 25, 1 (2005): 3–34.

128. Fontain, JR, Heo, M, Bathon, JM. Are US adults with arthritis meeting public health recommendations for physical activity? Arthritis & Rheumatism 50:624–628, 2004.

129. The American Journal of Clinical Nutrition 25: June1972, pp. 555–558. "Incidence of osteoporosis in vegetarians and omnivores."

130. Giem, P, Beeson, LW, Fraser, GE. Neuroepidemiology 1993;12:28–36. The Incidence of Dementia and Intake of Animal Products: Preliminary Findings from the Adventist Health Study.

131. "Position of the American Dietetic Association and Dietitians of Canada: Vegetarian diets." Journal of the American Dietetic Association, 2003, 06. Accessed 4 January 2007.

132. Key, TJ, Appleby, PN, Rosell, MS. "Health effects of vegetarian and vegan diets" (abstract). Proceedings of the Nutrition Society, 2006, 65:35–41. Accessed 4 January 2007.

133. Apple, PN, Thorogood, M, Mann, JI, Key, TJ. "The Oxford Vegetarian Study: an overview." American Journal of Clinical Nutrition, 1999, 70:525S–531S.

134. Jensen, MK, Koh-Benerjee, P, Hu, FB, Franz, M, Sampson L, Gronbaek, M, Rimm, EBSO. Intakes of whole grains, bran, and germ and the risk of coronary heart disease in men. Am J Clin Nutr 2004 Dec;80(6):1492–9.

135. Gillma, MW, Cupples, LA, Gagnon, D, Posner, BM, Ellison, RC, Castelli, WP, Wolf, PA. Protective effect of fruits and vegetables on development of stroke in men. SOJAMA 1995 Apr 12;273(14):1113–7.

136. Willett, WC. Diet and cancer: an evolving picture. JAMA 2005; 293:233.

137. Negri, E, Franceschi, S, Parpinel, M, La Vecchia, C. Fiber intake and risk of colorectal cancer. Cancer Epidemiol Biomarkers Prev 1998; 7:667.

138. National Library of Medicine (www.nlm.nih.gov/medlineplus/dietaryfiber.html).

139. National Institute on Diabetes and Digestive and Kidney Diseases (www.niddk.nih.gov)

140. Harvard School of Public Health (www.hsph.harvard.edu/nutritionsource/what-should-you- eat/fiber/index.html).

141. Sonestedt, E. The International Journal of Cancer 123 (7): 1637–1643.

142. http://www.sweetsurprise.com.

143. The Health Effects of High Fructose Syrup, Report 3 of The Council on Science and Public Health (A-08), The American Medical Association.

144. http://www.washingtonpost.com/wp-dyn/content/article/2009/01/26/AR2009012601831.html. Washington Post: Study Finds HFCS Contains Mercury Jan. 2009.

145. http://www.cbsnews.com/stories/2008/10/01/cbsnews_investigates/main4491513.shtml CBS News Investigates "Sweetener Controversy Grows" Oct. 2008.

146. http://stanford.wellsphere.com/parenting-article/high-fructose-corn-syrup-controversy/640342 Stanford. Wellsphere HFCS Controversy Apr. 2009.

147. Smith, A. Effects of caffeine on human behavior. Food Chem Toxicol 2002;40(9):1243–1255.

148. Rapuri, PB, Gallagher, JC, Kinyamu, HK, Ryschon, KL. Caffeine intake increases the rate of bone loss in elderly women and interacts with vitamin D receptor genotypes. Am J Clin Nutr 2001;74(6):694–700.

149. Shuh, KJ, Griffiths, RR. Caffeine reinforcement: The role of withdrawal. Psychopharmacology 1997;130(4):320–326.

150. Norager, CB, Jensen, MB, Madsen, MR, Laurberg, S. Caffeine improves endurance in 75-yr-ol citizens: A randomized, double-blind, placebocontrolled, crossover study. J Appl Physiol 2005;99(6):2302–2306.
151. Dodick, DW. Chronic daily headache. N Engl J Med 2006;354(2):158–165.
152. Delacretaz, E. Supraventricular tachycardia. N Engl J Med 2006;354(10):1039–1051. Silber MH. Chronic insomnia. N Engl J Med 2005;353(8):803–810.
153. Lantz, MS. Anxiety, Headaches, Insomnia, Restless Legs, and Hypertension: Multiple Disorders or One Problem? Clinical Geritatrics Volume 15 - Issue 4 - April 2007 Page: 16–19.
154. Harrington, S. Abstract The role of sugar-sweetened beverage consumption in adolescent obesity: a review of the literature. J Sch Nurs. 2008 Feb;24(1):3–12.
155. Ebbeling, CB, Feldman, HA, Osganian, SK, Chomitz, VR, Ellenbogen, SJ, Ludwig, DS. Free Full Text Effects of decreasing sugar-sweetened beverage consumption on body weight in adolescents: a randomized, controlled pilot study. Pediatrics. 2006 Mar;117(3):673–80.
156. Montonen, J, Ja"rvinen, R, Knekt, P, Helio"vaara, M, Reunanen, A. Abstract Consumption of sweetened beverages and intakes of fructose and glucose predict type 2 diabetes occurrence. J Nutr. 2007 Jun;137(6):1447–54.
157. Schulze, MB, Manson, JE, Ludwig, DS, Colditz, GA, Stampfer, MJ, Willett, WC, Hu, FB. Free Full Text Sugar-sweetened beverages, weight gain, and incidence of type 2 diabetes in young and middle-aged women. JAMA. 2004 Aug 25;292(8):927–34.
158. Tucker, KL, Morita, K, Qiao, N, Hannan, MT, Cupples, LA, Kiel, DP. Free Full Text Colas, but not other carbonated beverages, are associated with low bone mineral density in older women: The Framingham Osteoporosis Study. Am J Clin Nutr. 2006 Oct;84(4):936–42.
159. Kristensen, M, Jensen, M, Kudsk, J, Henriksen, M, Mølgaard, C. Abstract Short-term effects on bone turnover of replacing milk with cola beverages: a 10-day interventional study in young men. Osteoporos Int. 2005 Dec;16(12):1803–8. Epub 2005 May 11.
160. Ma, D, Jones, G. Soft drink and milk consumption, physical activity, bone mass, and upper limb fractures in children: a population-based case-control study. Calcif Tissue Int. 2004 Oct;75(4):286–91. Epub 2004 Jul 30.
161. http://www.webmd.com/oral-health/news/20040611/sodas-canned-teas-attack-tooth-enamel.
162. Weiss, GH, Sluss, PM, Linke, CA. Changes in urinary magnesium, citrate, and oxalate levels due to cola consumption. Urology. 1992 Apr;39(4):331–3.

163. Rodgers, A. Effect of cola consumption on urinary biochemical and physicochemical risk factors associated with calcium oxalate urolithiasis. Urol Res. 1999;27(1):77–81.

164. Saldana, TM, Basso, O, Darden, R, Sandler, DP. Abstract Carbonated beverages and chronic kidney disease. Epidemiology. 2007 Jul;18(4):501–6.

165. Brown, CM, Dulloo, AG, Yepuri, G, Montani, JP. Abstract Fructose ingestion acutely elevates blood pressure in healthy young humans.

166. Zelber-Sagi, S, Nitzan-Kaluski, D, Goldsmith, R, Webb, M, Blendis, L, Halpern, Z, Oren, R. Long term nutritional intake and the risk for non-alcoholic fatty liver disease (NAFLD): a population based study. J Hepatol. 2007 Nov;47(5):711–7.

167. http://news.ninemsn.com.au/article.aspx?id=269520 (Soft drink additive damages DNA: report Mon May 28 2007 National Nine News).

168. PLACE THE BMI CHART REFERENCE

169. http://apps.who.int/bmi/index.jsp?introPage=intro_3.html "International Classification of Weight based on BMI."

170. J Clin Invest. 1980 June; 65(6): 1272–1284. Mechanisms of insulin resistance in human obesity: evidence for receptor and postreceptor defects.

171. Obesity surgery 2003, vol. 13, no 5, pp. 699–705.

172. Carpenter, J, Carr, S, Hogan, J, Haydon, B, Somers, M, Robbins, L, Cowett, R. Insulin resistance in gestational diabetes: Effect of obesity American Journal of Obstetrics and Gynecology, January 1997, Volume 176, Issue 1, Pages S23–S23.

173. Current Opinion in Endocrinology & Diabetes:October 2001 - Volume 8 - Issue 5 - pp 235–239 Obesity and nutrition Obesity, free fatty acids, and insulin resistance.

174. http://www.sciencedaily.com/releases/2007/04/070404162428.htm (Dieting Does Not Work, Researchers Report. ScienceDaily).

175. http://www.atkinsexposed.org/atkins/79/American_Kidney_Fund.htm. "AKF Warns About Impact of High-Protein Diets On Kidney Health."

176. http://www.kidney.org/professionals/kdoqi/guidelines_bp/guide_6.htm. Guideline 6: Dietary and Other Therapeutic Lifestyle Changes in Adults.

177. http://www.kidney.org/professionals/kdoqi/guideline_diabetes/guide5. htm. "Guideline 5: Nutritional Management in Diabetes and Chronic Kidney Disease."

178. http://www.fwhc.org/health/high-protein-diet.htm.

179. McCay, CM, Crowel, MF, Maynard, LA. (1935) The effect of retarded growth upon the length of the life span and upon the ultimate body size. J Nutr 10: 63–79.

180. Weindruch, R, Walford, RL. (1988) The retardation of aging and disease by dietary restriction. Springfield (Illinois): Charles C. Thomas. 436 p.

181. Bodkin, NL, Alexander, TM, Ortmeyer, HK, Johnson, E, Hansen, BC. (2003) Mortality and morbidity in laboratory-maintained Rhesus monkeys and effects of long-term dietary restriction. J Gerontol A Biol Sci Med Sci 58: 212–219. Find this article online

182. Lane, MA, Black, A, Ingram, DK, Roth, GS. (1998) Calorie restriction in non-human primates: implications for age-related disease risk. J Anti-Aging Med 1: 315–326. Find this article online

183. http://www.win.niddk.nih.gov/publications/myths.htm.

184. Berquin, IM. "Modulation of prostate cancer genetic risk by omega-3 and omega-6 fatty acids." The Journal of Clinical Investigation 117 (7): 1866–75.

185. Mensink, RP. "Dietary saturated and trans fatty acids and lipoprotein metabolism." Annals of Medicine 26 (6): 461–4.

186. Idris, CA. "Effect of dietary cholesterol, trans and saturated fatty acids on serum lipoproteins in non-human primates." Asia Pacific Journal of Clinical Nutrition 11 (Suppl 7): S408–15.

187. Jonnalagadda, SS. "Dietary fats rich in saturated fatty acids enhance gallstone formation relative to monounsaturated fat in cholesterol-fed hamsters." Lipids 30 (5): 415–24.

188. Kromhout, D. "Dietary saturated and trans fatty acids and cholesterol and 25-year mortality from coronary heart disease: the Seven Countries Study." Preventive Medicine 24 (3): 308–15.

189. Khosla, P, Hajri, T. "Decreasing dietary lauric and myristic acids improves plasma lipids more favorably than decreasing dietary palmitic acid in rhesus monkeys fed AHA step 1 type diets." The Journal of Nutrition 127 (3): 525S–530S.

190. Nicolosi, RJ. (May 1997). "Dietary fat saturation effects on low-density-lipoprotein concentrations and metabolism in various animal models." The American Journal of Clinical Nutrition 65 (5 Suppl): 1617S–1627S.

191. Stewart-Phillips, JL. "Genetically determined susceptibility and resistance to diet-induced atherosclerosis in inbred strains of mice." The Journal of Laboratory and Clinical Medicine 112 (1): 36–42.

192. Nikkari, ST. "The hyperlipidemic hamster as an atherosclerosis model." Artery 18 (6): 285–90.

193. Otto, J. "Lovastatin inhibits diet induced atherosclerosis in F1B golden Syrian hamsters." Atherosclerosis 114 (1): 19–28.

194. Kowala, MC. "Regression of early atherosclerosis in hyperlipidemic hamsters induced by fosinopril and captopril." Journal of Cardiovascular Pharmacology 25 (2): 179–

195. http://en.wikipedia.org/wiki/Vegetable_fats_and_oils.

196. Hollis, JH, Mattes, RD. Effect of chronic consumption of almonds on body weight in healthy humans. Br J Nutr. 2007;98:651–6.

197. Wien, MA, Sabate, J, Ikle, DN, Cole, SE, Kandeel, FR. Almonds vs. complex carbohydrates in a weight reduction program. Int J Obes Relat Metab Disord. 2003;27:1365–72.

198. Alper, CM, Mattes, RD. The effects of chronic peanut consumption on energy balance and hedonics. Int J Obes. 2002;26:1129–37.

199. Alasalvar, C, Shahidi, F. Tree Nuts: Composition, Phytochemicals, and Health Effects (Nutraceutical Science and Technology). CRC. pp. 143.

200. Black, M, Halmer, P. (2006). The encyclopedia of seeds: science, technology and uses. Wallingford, UK: CABI. p. 228.

201. http://en.wikipedia.org/wiki/Nut_(fruit)the_encyclopedia_of_seeds-1.

202. Kelly, JH. Nuts and coronary heart disease: an epidemiological perspective. Br J Nutr 96, S61–S67.

203. Sabaté, J. Effects of walnuts on serum lipid levels and blood pressure in normal men. N Engl J Med 328, 603–607.

204. Josse, AR. Almonds and postprandial glycemia—a dose response study. Metabolism, 56, 400–404.

205. Fraser, GE. Ten years of life: Is it a matter of choice? Arch Int Med, 161, 1645–1652 (2001).

206. Sabaté, J. Walnuts and fatty fish influence different serum lipid fractions in normal to mildly hyperlipidemic individuals: a randomized controlled study. Am J Clin Nutr 2009, 89, 1657S–1663S.

207. Salas-Salvadó, J, et al. Effect of a Mediterranean diet supplemented with nuts on metabolic syndrome status: one-year results of the PREDIMED randomized trial. Archives of Internal Medicine 168:2449–58 (2008).

208. Kushi, L. Dietary antioxidant vitamins and death from coronary heart disease in post-menopausal women. New England Journal of Medicine 334:1156–62 (1996).

209. Hu, FB. Frequent nut consumption and risk of coronary heart disease in women. British Medical Journal 317:1341–5 (1998).

210. Albert, CM. Nut consumption and decreased risk of sudden cardiac death in the physicians' health study. Archives of Internal Medicine 162:1382–7 (2002).

211. Fraser, GE. Effect of risk factor values on lifetime risk of and age at first coronary event. The Adventist Health Study. American Journal of Epidemiology 142:746–58 (1995).

212. Yochum, LA. Intake of antioxidant vitamins and risk of death from stroke in post-menopausal women. American Journal of Clinical Nutrition 72: 476–483 (2000).

213. Jiang, R. Nut and peanut butter consumption and risk of type 2 diabetes in women. Journal of the American Medical Association 288: 2554–2560 (2002).

214. Hernan, MA. Intakes of vitamins E and C, carotenoids, vitamin supplements, and PD risk. Neurology 59:1161–9 (2002).

215. Seddon, JM. Progression of age-related macular degeneration: association with dietary fat, transunsaturated fat, nuts and fish intake. Archives of Ophthalmology 121:1728–37 (2003).

216. Tsai, CJ. Frequent nut consumption and decreased risk of cholecystectomy in women. American Journal of Clinical Nutrition 80:76–81 (2004).

217. Hu, FB. Nut consumption and risk of coronary heart disease: a review of the epidemiologic evidence. Current Atherosclerosis Reports 1:204–209 (1999).

218. Jiang, R. Nut and peanut butter consumption and risk of type 2 diabetes in women. Journal of the American Medical Association 288: 2554–2560 (2002).

219. Sabaté, J. Nut consumption, vegetarian diets, ischemic heart disease risk, and all-cause mortality: evidence from epidemiologic studies. American Journal of Clinical Nutrition 70 (Suppl):500S–3S (1999).

220. Berquin, IM. "Modulation of prostate cancer genetic risk by omega-3 and omega-6 fatty acids." The Journal of Clinical Investigation 117 (7): 1866–75.

221. http://www.ivu.org/faq/nutrition.html.

222. www.vegetarian.org.uk.

223. www.vegetarian.org.uk/adverts.html.

224. http://www.mypyramid.gov/pyramid/index.html.

225. Groff, J, Gropper, S. Advanced Nutrition and Human Metabolism, 3rd ed. Wadsworth: 2000.

226. Herbert, V. Vitamin B-12: plant sources, requirements, and assay. Am J Clin Nutr. 1988;48:852–8.

227. Hathcock, JN, Troendle, GJ. Oral cobalamin for treatment of pernicious anemia? JAMA. 1991 Jan 2;265(1):96–7.

228. Crane, MG, Sample, C, Pathcett, S, Register, UD. "Vitamin B12 studies in total vegetarians (vegans). Journal of Nutritional Medicine. 1994;4:419–430.

229. Herbert, V. (September 1988). "Vitamin B-12: plant sources, requirements, and assay." The American Journal of Clinical Nutrition 48 (3 Suppl): 852–8.

230. http://www.ajcn.org/cgi/pmidlookup?view=long&pmid=3046314.

231. Jaouen, G, ed. (2006). Bioorganometallics: Biomolecules, Labeling, Medicine. Weinheim: Wiley- VCH.

232. Loeffler, G. (2005). Basiswissen Biochemie. Heidelberg: Springer. p. 606. ISBN 3-540-23885-9.

233. Khan, AG, Eswaran, SV. (2003). "Woodward's synthesis of vitamin B12." Resonance 8: 8.

234. Eschenmoser, A, Wintner, CE. (June 1977). "Natural product synthesis and vitamin B12." Science 196 (4297): 1410–20

235. Butler, RN, Davis, R, Lewis, CB, et al. Physical fitness: benefits of exercising for the older patient. Geriatrics 53(10):46–62. 1998.

236. American Heart Association. 2002 heart and stroke statistical update. Dallas, TX: American Heart Association, 2001.

237. Centers for Disease Control and Prevention. National diabetes fact sheet: general information and national estimates on diabetes in the United States, 2000. Atlanta, GA: US Department of Health and Human Services, Centers for Disease Control and Prevention, 2002.

238. American Cancer Society. Cancer facts & figures 2002. Atlanta, GA: American Cancer Society. Inc., 2002.

239. Vainio, H, Bianchini, F, eds. Weight control and physical activity. IARC Handbooks of Cancer Prevention. IARC Press Vol 6, 2002.

240. McGinnis, JM, Foege, WH. Actual causes of death in the United States. JAMA 270(18):207–12. 1993.

241. Hahn, RA, Teuesch, SM, Rothenberg, RB, et al. Excess deaths from nine chronic diseases in the United States, 1986. JAMA 264(20):2554–59. 1998.

242. Paffenbarger, RS, Hyde, RT, Wing, AL, et al. The association of changes in physical–activity level and other lifestyle characteristics with mortality among men. N Engl J Med 328(8):538–45. 1993.

243. Sherman, SE, D'Agostino, RB, Cobb, JL, et al. Physical activity and mortality in women in the Framingham Heart Study. Am Heart J 128(5):879–84. 1994.

244. Kaplan, GAA, Strawbridge, WJ, Cohen, RD, et al. Natural history of leisure-time physical activity and its correlates: Associations with mortality from all causes and cardiovascular diseases over 28 years. Am J Epid 144(8):793–97. 1996.

245. Kushi, LH, Fee, RM, Folsom, AR, et al. Physical activity and mortality in postmenopausal women. JAMA 277:1287–92. 1997.

246. Lee, CD, Blair, SN, Jackson, AS. Cardiorespiratory fitness, body composition, and all-cause and cardiovascular disease mortality in men. Am J Clin Nutr 69 (3):373–80. 1999.

247. Wei, M, Kampert, JB, Barlow, CE, et al. Relationship between low cardiorespiratory fitness and mortality in normal-weight, overweight, and obese men. JAMA 282(16):1547–53. 1999.

248. US Department of Health and Human Services. Leisure-time physical activity among adults: United States, 1997–98. US Department of Health and Human Services, Centers for Disease Control and Prevention, National Center for Health Statistics, 2002.

249. Centers for Disease Control and Prevention. CDC Surveillance Summaries, December 17, 1999. MMWR 48(no. SS-8). 1999.

250. Kann, L, et al. Youth risk behavior surveillance–United States, 1999. In: CDC Surveillance Summaries, June 9, 2000. MMWR 49(No. SS-5):1–96. 2000.

251. Warburton, DER, Nicol, CW, Bredin, SSD. Canadian Medical Association Journal (CMAJ) • March 14, 2006; 174 (6). Health benefits of physical activity: the evidence.

252. Smith, GD, Frankel, S, Yarnell, J. Sex and death: are they related? Findings from the Caerphilly cohort study BMJ 1997;315:1641–1644 (20 December).

253. http://www.forbes.com/2003/10/08/cz_af_1008health.html 'Is Sex necessary'.

254. http://www.cnn.com/2010/HEALTH/01/07/sex.health.benefits/index.html.

255. http://www.financialnewsusa.com/more/56-living-health/10729-sex-can-lead-to-healthier-life.

256. Doheny, K. (2008) "10 Surprising Health Benefits of Sex," WebMD (reviewed by Chang, L., M.D.) Patti Britton, PhD, president, American Association of Sexuality Educators and Therapists.

257. Ogden, G. sex therapist and marriage and family therapist, Cambridge, Mass. Joy Davidson, PhD, psychologist and sex therapist, author, Fearless Sex.

258. http://www.cnn.com/2010/HEALTH/01/07/sex.health.benefits/index.html.

259. http://www.webmd.com/sex-relationships/features/10-surprising-health-benefits-of-sex.

260. Brody, S. (2006). Blood pressure reactivity to stress is better for people who recently had penile- vaginal intercourse than for people who had other or no sexual activity. Biological Psychology, 71, 214–222.

261. Leitzmann, MF, Platz, EA, Stamper, MJ, Willett, WC, Giovannucci, E. Ejaculation Frequency and Subsequent Risk of Prostate Cancer JAMA. 2004;291:1578–1586.

262. http://www.advancednaturalmedicine.com/prostate-health-and-ejaculation.html.

263. Brody, S, Fischer, AH, Hess, U. (2008). Women's finger sensitivity correlates with partnered sexual behavior but not solitary masturbation frequencies. Journal of Sex & Marital Therapy, in press.

264. Brody, S. (2007). Intercourse orgasm consistency, concordance of women's genital and subjective sexual arousal, and erotic stimulus presentation sequence. Journal of Sex & Marital Therapy, 33, 31–39.

265. Brody, S. (2007). Vaginal orgasm is associated with better psychological function. Sexual & Relationship Therapy, 22, 173–191.

266. Costa, RM, Brody S. (2007). Women's relationship quality is associated with specifically penile-vaginal intercourse orgasm and frequency. Journal of Sex & Marital Therapy, 33, 319–327.

267. Hess, U, Brody, S, Van Der Schalk, J, Fischer, AH. (2007). Sexual activity is inversely related to women's perceptions of the facial attractiveness of unknown men. Personality and Individual Differences, 43, 1991–1997.

268. Brody, S. (2006). Penile-vaginal intercourse is better: Evidence trumps ideology. Sexual & Relationship Therapy, 21, 393–403.

269. Brody, S. (2006). Blood pressure reactivity to stress is better for people who recently had penile- vaginal intercourse than for people who had other or no sexual activity. Biological Psychology, 71, 214–222.

270. Brody, S, Krüger, THC. (2006). The post-orgasmic prolactin increase following intercourse is greater than following masturbation and suggests greater satiety. Biological Psychology, 71, 312–315.

271. Brody, S, Potterat, JJ, Muth, SQ, Woodhouse, DE. (2005). Psychiatric and characterological factors relevant to excess mortality in a long-term cohort of prostitute women. Journal of Sex & Marital Therapy, 31, 97–112.

272. Brody, S. (2004). Sexual factors and prostate cancer. BJU International: British Journal of Urology, 93, 180.

273. Brody, S. (2004). Slimness is associated with greater intercourse and lesser masturbation frequency. Journal of Sex & Marital Therapy, 30, 251–261.

274. Brody, S, Keller, U, Degen, L, Cox, DJ, Schächinger, H. (2004). Selective processing of food words during insulin induced hypoglycemia in healthy humans. Psychopharmacology, 173, 217–220.

275. Nava, E, Landau, D, Brody, S, Schächinger, H. (2004). Relaxation increases parasympathetic activity and improves incidental memory. Neurobiology of Learning and Memory, 81, 167–171.

276. Potterat, JJ, Brewer, D, Muth, SW, Rothenberg, RB, Woodhouse, DE, Muth, JB, Stites, HK, Brody, S. (2004). Mortality in a long-term open cohort of prostitute women. American Journal of Epidemiology, 159, 778–785.

277. Potterat, JJ, Gisselquist, D, Brody, S. (2004). Still not understanding the uneven spread of HIV within Africa. Sexually Transmitted Diseases, 31, 365.

278. Schächinger, H, Port, J, Brody, S, Linder, L, Wilhelm, F, Huber, PR, Cox, D, Keller, U. (2004). Increased high-frequency heart rate variability during insulin-induced hypoglycemia in healthy humans. Clinical Science, 106, 583–588.

279. Brody, S. (2003). Exercise intensity and risk of coronary heart disease. JAMA: Journal of the American Medical Association, 289, 419.

280. Brody, S. (2003). Alexithymia is inversely associated with women's frequency of vaginal intercourse. Archives of Sexual Behavior, 32, 73–77.

281. Brody, S, Laan, E, van Lunsen, RHW. (2003). Concordance between women's physiological and subjective sexual arousal is associated with consistency of orgasm during intercourse but not other sexual behavior. Journal of Sex & Marital Therapy, 29, 15–23.

282. Brody, S, Preut, R. (2003). Vaginal intercourse frequency and heart rate variability. Journal of Sex & Marital Therapy, 29, 371–380.

283. Schächinger, H, Cox, D, Linder, L, Brody, S, Keller, U. (2003). Cognitive and psychomotor function in hypoglycemia: Response error patterns and retest reliability. Pharmacology, Biochemistry and Behavior, 75, 915–920.

284. http://www.betterhealth.vic.gov.au/bhcv2/bhcarticles.nsf/pages/Kissing_and_your_health.

285. http://soundmedicine.iu.edu/segment/53/Health-Benefits-of-Kissing.

286. http://www.articlesbase.com/mens-health-articles/5-tips-to-improve-your-marriage-with-love- making-2498769.html.

287. http://www.healthdiscovery.net/links/calculators/calorie_calculator.htm.

288. http://ezinearticles.com/?How-Many-Calories-Are-Burned-During-Sex?&id=4392523.

289. http://mayoresearch.mayo.edu/levine_lab/about.cfm.

290. Levine, JA. Non-exercise activity thermogenesis (NEAT).Best Pract Res Clin Endocrinol Metab. 2002 Dec;16(4):679–702.

291. Levine, JA. Nonexercise activity thermogenesis (NEAT): environment and biology. Am J Physiol Endocrinol Metab. 2004 May;286(5):E675–85.

292. Levine, JA. "Non-Exercise Activity Thermogenesis." Mayo Clinic. 2010.

293. Vaccariello, L. "7 Easy Ways to Lose Weight Without Starving or Breaking a Sweat." Prevention. Health.Yahoo.com 2010.

294. Blackburn, G. (1995). Effect of degree of weight loss on health benefits. Obesity Research 3: 211S–216S.

295. NIH, NHLBI Obesity Education Initiative. Clinical Guidelines on the Identification, Evaluation, and Treatment of Overweight and Obesity in Adults.

296. http://www.cdc.gov/healthyweight/losing_weight/index.html.

297. "Statistics Related to Overweight and Obesity." CDC. 2006. http://www. win.niddk.nih.gov/statistics. Retrieved 2009-01-23.

298. http://web.archive.org/web/20060206185213/www.naaso.org/statistics/ obesity_trends.asp. Retrieved 2008-03-08. "Obesity Statistics: U.S. Obesity Trends." North American Association for the Study of Obesity. 2006.

299. http://www.cdc.gov/nchs/data/nhis/earlyrelease/200506_06.pdf, retrieved 2008-03-15. Early Release of Selected Estimates Based on Data From the 2004 National Health Interview Survey, CDC NCHS, 2005-06-21.

300. http://www.cdc.gov/healthyweight/losing_weight/index.html.

301. http://www.americanheart.org/presenter.jhtml?identifier=4639.

302. Wachman, A, Bernstein, DS. "Diet and osteoporosis" Lancet 1968 1:958.

303. Ellis, FR, et al. "Incidence of osteoporosis in vegetarians and omnivores" American Journal of Clinical Nutrition, June 1972, 25:555–558

304. Mazess, RB, Mather, W. "Bone mineral content of North Alaskan Eskimos" American Journal of Clinical Nutrition, September 1974 2:916–925.

305. Spencer, H, Kramer, L. "Factors contributing to osteoporosis," Journal of Nutrition, 1986 116:316–319.

306. Spencer, H, Kramer, L. "Further studies of the effect of a high protein diet as meat on calcium metabolism," American Journal of Clinical Nutrition, June 1983 37 (6):924–929..

307. Linkswiler, HM, et al. "Calcium retention of young adult males as affected by level or protein and of caclcium intake", Trans. N.Y. Acad. Sci, 1974 36:333.

308. Spencer, H., et al. "Do Protein and Phosphorus Cause Calcium Loss?" American Institute of Nutrition, 1988:657–660.

309. Meyer, TW, Anderson, SA, Rennke, HG, Brenner, BM. Reversing glomerular hypertension stabilizes established glomerular injury. Kidney Int 1987; 31:752.

310. Zatz, R, Meyer, TW, Rennke, HG, Brenner, BM. Predominance of hemodynamic rather than metabolic factors in the pathogenesis of diabetic nephropathy. Proc Natl Acad Sci USA 1985; 82:5963.

311. Miller, PL, Scholey, JW, Rennke, HG, Meyer, TW. Glomerular hypertrophy aggravates epithelial cell injury in nephrotic rats. J Clin Invest 1990; 85:1119.

312. Fukui, M, Nakamura, T, Ebihara, I, et al. Low-protein diet attenuates increased gene expression of platelet-derived growth factor and transforming growth factor-ß in experimental glomerular sclerosis. J Lab Clin Med 1993; 121:224.

313. Nakamura, T, Fukui, M, Ebihara, I, et al. Low protein diet blunts the rise in glomerular gene expression in focal glomerulosclerosis. Kidney Int 1994; 45:1593.

314. Woods, LL. Mechanisms of renal hemodynamic regulation in response to protein feeding. Kidney Int 1993; 44:659.

315. King, AJ, Levey, AS. Dietary protein and renal function. J Am Soc Nephrol 1993; 3:1723.

316. Nakamura, H, Ho, S, Ebe, N, Shibata, A. Renal effects of different types of proteins in healthy volunteers and diabetic patients. Diabetes Care 1993; 16:1071.

317. Kontessis, P, Jones, S, Dodds, R, et al. Renal, metabolic and hormonal responses to ingestion of animal and vegetable proteins. Kidney Int 1990; 38:136.

318. Schriner, SE, Linford, NJ, Martin, GM, Treuting, P, Ogburn, CE, Emond, M, Coskun, PE, Ladiges, W, Wolf, N, Van Remmen, H, Wallace, DC, Rabinovitch, PS. (2005). "Extension of murine life span by overexpression of catalase targeted to mitochondria." Science 308 (5730): 1909–11.

319. de Magalhaes, JP, Church, GM. (2006). "Cells discover fire: employing reactive oxygen species in development and consequences for aging." Exp Gerontol 41(1):1–10.

320. de Magalhaes, JP, Costa, J, Church, GM. (2007). "An analysis of the relationship between metabolism, developmental schedules, and longevity using phylogenetic independent contrasts." J Gerontol A Biol Sci Med Sci 62(2):149–160.

321. Dierick, Frippiat, Salmon, Chainiaux, and Toussaint (2003). "Cells, stress and tissue ageing." In: Biology of Aging and its Modulation, Rattan, S. I. S. (ed.). Kluwer, Amsterdam, 101–125.

322. DiMauro, S, Tanji, K, Bonilla, E, Pallotti, F, Schon, EA. (2002). "Mitochondrial abnormalities in muscle and other aging cells: classification, causes, and effects." Muscle Nerve 26(5):597–607.

323. Dimauro, S, Schon, EA. (2003). "Mitochondrial respiratory-chain diseases." N Engl J Med 348(26):2656–2668. PubMed.

324. http://www.senescence.info.

325. Kushi, LH, Byers, T, Doyle, C, Bandera, EV, McCullough, M, McTiernan, A, Gansler, T, Andrews, KS, Thun, MJ. American Cancer Society 2006 Nutrition and Physical Activity Guidelines Advisory Committee. American Cancer Society guidelines on Nutrition and Physical Activity for cancer prevention: reducing the risk of cancer with healthy food choices and physical activity. CA Cancer J Clin. 2006;56:254–281.

326. Campbell, JK, Canene-Adams, K, Lindshield, BL, Boileau, TW, Clinton, SK, Erdman, JW Jr. Tomato phytochemicals and prostate cancer risk. J Nutr. 2004; 134:3486S–3492S.

327. Clark, PE, Hall, MC, Borden, LS Jr., et al. Phase I–II prospective dose-escalating trial of lycopene in patients with biochemical relapse of prostate cancer after definitive local therapy. Urology.2006;67:1257–1261.

328. Doyle, C, Kushi, LH, Byers, T, et al. The 2006 Nutrition, Physical Activity and Cancer Survivorship Advisory Committee. American Cancer Society. Nutrition and physical activity during and after cancer treatment: an American Cancer Society guide for informed choices. CA: a Cancer Journal for Clinicians. 2006;56:323–353.

329. Etminan, M, Takkouche, B, Caamano-Isorna, F. The role of tomato products and lycopene in the prevention of prostate cancer: a meta-analysis of observational studies. Cancer Epidemiol Biomarkers Prev. 2004;13:340–345.

330. Gerster, H. The potential role of lycopene for human health. J Am Coll Nutr. 1997;16:109–126.

331. Giovannucci, E. Tomatoes, tomato-based products, lycopene, and cancer: review of the epidemiologic literature. J Natl Cancer Inst. 1999;91:317–331.

332. Goodman, M, Bostick, RM, Ward, KC, et al. Lycopene intake and prostate cancer risk: effect modification by plasma antioxidants and the XRCC1 genotype. Nutrition & Cancer. 2006;55:13–20.

333. Jatoi, A, Burch, P, Hillman, D, et al. A tomato-based, lycopene-containing intervention for androgen- independent prostate cancer: results of a Phase II study from the North Central Cancer Treatment Group. Urology. 2007;69:289–294.

334. Kirsh, VA, Mayne, ST, Peters, U, et al. A prospective study of lycopene and tomato product intake and risk of prostate cancer. Cancer Epidemiology, Biomarkers & Prevention. 2006;15:92–98.

335. Kushi, LH, Byers, T, Doyle, C, et al. American Cancer Society Guidelines on Nutrition and Physical Activity for cancer prevention: reducing the risk of cancer with healthy food choices and physical activity. CA: a Cancer Journal for Clinicians.2006;56:254–281.

336. Angerer, P, von Schacky, C. n-3 polyunsaturated fatty acids and the cardiovascular system. Curr Opin Lipidol. 2000;11(1):57–63.

337. Hooper, L, Thompson, R, Harrison, R, et al. Omega 3 fatty acids for prevention and treatment of cardiovascular disease. Cochrane Database Syst Rev. 2004;CD003177.

338. Iso, H, Rexrode, KM, Stampfer, MJ, Manson, JE, Colditz, GA, Speizer, FE, et al. Intake of fish and omega-3 fatty acids and risk of stroke in women. JAMA. 2001;285(3):304–312.

339. Galli, C, Risé, P. Fish consumption, omega 3 fatty acids and cardiovascular disease. The science and the clinical trials. Nutr Health. 2009;20(1):11–20. Review.

340. Ramírez–Tortosa, MC. Oral administration of a turmeric extract inhibits LDL oxidation and has hypocholesterolemic effects in rabbits with experimental atherosclerosis. Atherosclerosis. 1999 Dec;147(2):371–8.

341. Davis, JM, Murphy, EA, Carmichael, MD, Zielinski, MR, Groschwitz, CM, Brown, AS, Ghaffar, A, Mayer, EP. Curcumin effects on inflammation and performance recovery following eccentric exercise-induced muscle damage. Am J Physiol Regul Integr Comp Physiol. 2007 Mar 1.

342. Dorai, T, Cao, YC, Dorai, B, Buttyan, R, Katz, AE. Therapeutic potential of curcumin in human prostate cancer. III. Curcumin inhibits proliferation, induces apoptosis, and inhibits angiogenesis of LNCaP prostate cancer cells in vivo. Prostate. 2001;47(4):293–303.

343. Dorai, T, Gehani, N, Katz, A. Therapeutic potential of curcumin in human prostate cancer. II. Curcumin inhibits tyrosine kinase activity of epidermal growth factor receptor and depletes the protein. Mol Urol. 2000;4(1):1–6.

344. Funk, JL, Frye, JB, Oyarzo, JN, Kuscuoglu, N, Wilson, J, McCaffrey, G, et al. Efficacy and mechanism of action of turmeric supplements in the treatment of experimental arthritis. Arthritis Rheum. 2006 Nov;54(11):3452–64.

345. Gautam, SC, Gao, X, Dulchavsky, S. Immunodilation by curcumin. Adv Exp Med Biol. 2007;595:321–41.

346. Gescher, AJ, Sharma, RA, Steward, WP. Cancer chemoprevention by dietary constituents: a tale of failure and promise. Lancet Oncol. 2001;2(6):371–379.

347. Goel, A, Kunnumakkara, AB, Aggarwal, BB. Curcumin as "Curecumin": from kitchen to clinic. Biochem Pharmacol. 2008;75(4):787–809.

348. Hanai, H, Iida, T, Takeuchi, K, Watanabe, F, Maruyama, Y, Andoh, A, et al. Curcumin maintenance therapy for ulcerative colitis: randomized, multicenter, double-blind, placebo-controlled trial. Clin Gastroenterol Hepatol. 2006 Dec;4(12):1502–6.

349. Handler, N, Jaeger, W, Puschacher, H, Leisser, K, Erker, T. Synthesis of novel curcumin analogues and their evaluation as selective cyclooxygenase-1 (COX-1) inhibitors. Chem Pharm Bull (Tokyo). 2007 Jan;55(1):64–71.

350. Heck, AM, DeWitt, BA, Lukes, AL. Potential interactions between alternative therapies and warfarin. Am J Health Syst Pharm. 2000;57(13):1221–1227.

351. Jagetia, GC, Aggarwal, BB. "Spicing up" of the immune system by curcumin. J Clin Immunol. 2007;27(1):19–35.

352. Giuseppe, R. Journal of Nutrition, September 2008; pp 1939–1945 News release, Catholic University.

353. http://www.webmd.com/heart-disease/news/20080925/dark-chocolate-prevents-heart-disease.

354. http://hiqnews.megafoundation.org/cancer_prevention_diets.htm.

355. http://www.sciencedaily.com/releases/2001/10/011024073452.htm.

356. http://www.rps.psu.edu/probing/healthychocolate.html.

357. www.mit.edu/people/jeffrey/HarrisVARept97.pdf.

358. Criqui, MH, Ringel, BL. Does diet or alcohol explain the French paradox? Lancet .1994;344:1719–1723.

359. de Jong, HJ, de Goede, J, Oude Griep, LM, Geleijnse, JM. Alcohol consumption and blood lipids in elderly coronary patients. Metabolism. 2008 Sep;57(9):1286–92.

360. de Lorgeril, M, Salen, P, Martin, JL, Boucher, F, de Leiris, J. Interactions of wine drinking with omega-3 fatty acids in patients with coronary heart disease: a fish-like effect of moderate wine drinking. Am Heart J. 2008 Jan;155(1):175–81. Epub 2007 Sep 27.

361. Doll, R, Peto, R, Hall, E, et al. Mortality in relation to consumption of alcohol: 13 years' observations on male British doctors. British Med J . 1994;309:911–918.

362. Duncan, BB, Chambless, LE, Schmidt, MI, et al. Association of waist-to-hip ratio is different with wine than with beer or hard liquor consumption. Am J Epidemiol. 1995;142:1034–1038.

363. Friedman, GD, Klatsky, AL. Is alcohol good for your health? New Engl. J. Med. 1993;329:1882–1883.

364. Gronbaek, M, Deis, A, Sorensen, TIA, et al. Mortality associated with moderate intake of wine, beer, or spirits. British Med J .1995; 310:1165–1169.

365. Hennekens, CH, Willett, W, Rosner, B, et al. Effects of beer, wine, and liquor in coronary deaths. JAMA. 1979;242: 1973–1974.

366. Ira, J, Goldberg, MD, Mosca, L, et al. Wine and your heart—a science advisory for healthcare professionals from the Nutrition Committee,

Council on Epidemiology and Prevention, and Council on Cardiovascular Nursing of the American Heart Association. Circulation. 2001; 103:472–475.

367. Klatsky, AL. Drink to your health? Sci Am . 2003;288(2):74–81.
368. Klatsky, AL, Friedman, GD, Armstrong, MA, et al. Wine, liquor, beer, and mortality. Am J Epidemiol. 2003;158(6):585–95.
369. www.cdc.gov/alcohol/faqs.htm.
370. http://www.acg.gi.org/patients/cgp/cgpvol1.asp.
371. http://digestive.niddk.nih.gov/ddiseases/pubs/smoking.
372. Fatal poisoning from sodium phosphate enema (Martin) JAMA 1987;257:2190–2.
373. The case against colonic irrigation (Kizer) California Morbidity 38, September 27, 1985.
374. An outbreak of amebiasis spread by colonic irrig at a chiro clinic (Istre) New Engl J Med 1982;307:339–42.
375. Deaths related to coffee enemas (Eisele) JAMA 1980;244:1608–9.
376. The doctor is in--jail (Ballentine) FDA Consumer October 1981, pp. 30–1.
377. Strum, R. The effects of obesity, smoking and problem drinking on chronic medical problems and health care costs. Health Affairs 21(2):245–253. 2002.
378. http://www.cancer.org/docroot/ped/content/ped_10_2x_questions_about_smoking_tobacco_and_heal th.asp.
379. http://www.cdc.gov/tobacco/data_statistics/fact_sheets/health_effects/effects_cig_smoking.
380. www.cdc.gov/alcohol/faqs.htm.
381. Young, LR, Nestle, M. The contribution of expanding portion sizes to the U.S. obesity epidemic. Amer J Pub Health, 2002;92(2):246–249.
382. Nielsen, SJ, Popkin, BM. Patterns and trends in food portion sizes, 1977–1998. JAMA 2003;289(4):450–453.
383. Smiciklas-Wright, H, Mitchell, DC, Mickle, SJ, Goldman, JD, Cook, A. Foods commonly eaten in the United States, 1989–1991 and 1994–1996: are portion sizes changing? J Am Dietetic A 2003;103(1):41–47.
384. Rolls, BJ, Morris, EL, Roe, LS. Portion size of food affects energy intake in normal-weight and overweight men and women. Am J Clin Nutr 2002;76:1207–1213.
385. Rolls, BJ, Roe, LS, Meengs, JS, Wall, DE. Increasing the portion size of a sandwich increases energy intake. J Am Diet Assoc 2004;104:367–372.
386. Diliberti, N, Bordi, PL, Conklin, MT, Rolls, BR. Increased portion size leads to increased energy intake in a restaurant meal. Obesity Res 2004;12:562–568.

387. Pudel, VE, Oetting, M. Eating in the laboratory: behavioral aspects of the positive energy balance. Int J Obesity 1977;1:369–386.

388. Rolls, BJ, Roe, LS, Kral, TVE, Meengs, JS, Wall, DE. Increasing the portion size of a packaged snack increases energy intake in men and women. Appetite 2004;42(1)63–69.

389. Wansink, B, Park, SB. At the movies: how external cues and perceived taste impact consumption volume. J Database Marketing. 1996;60:1–14.

390. Fisher, JO, Rolls, BJ, Birch, LL. Children's bite size and intake of an entrée are greater with large portions than with age-appropriate or self-selected portions. Amer J Clin Nutr 2003;77(5):1164–1170.

391. Rolls, BJ, Engell, D, Birch, LL. Serving portion size influences 5-year-old but not 3-year-old children's food intakes. J Am Diet Assoc. 2000;1000:232–234.

392. McConahy, KL, Smiciklas-Wright, H, Birth, LL, Mitchell, DC, Picciano MF. Food portions are positively related to energy intake and body weight in early childhood. J Pediatr 2002;140(3):340–347.

393. McConahy, KL, Smiciklas-Wright, H, Mitchell, DC, Picciano, MF. Portion size of common foods predicts energy intake among preschool-aged children. J Amer Diet Assoc. 2004;104(6):975–979.

394. Rolls, BJ, Morris, EL, Roe, LS. Portion size of food affects energy intake in normal-weight and overweight men and women. Am J Clin Nutr 2002;76:1207–1213.

395. Young, LR, Nestle, MS. Portion sizes in dietary assessment: issues and policy implications. Nutr Rev 1995;53:149–158.

396. Ello-Martin, JA, Roe, LS, Meengs, JS, Wall, DE, Rolls, BJ. Increasing the portion size of a unit food increases energy intake. Appetite 2002;39:74.

397. Young, LR, Nestle, M. Variation in perceptions of a "medium" food portion: implications for dietary guidance. J Am Diet Assoc 1998;98:458–459.

398. Rolls, BJ. The supersizing of America: portion size and the obesity epidemic. Nutr Today 2003;38(2):42–53.

399. de la Torre, R, Pichini, S. Usefulness of Sweat Testing for the Detection of Cannabis Smoke Clinical Chemistry. 2004;50:1961–1962..

400. Caplan, YH, Goldberger, BA. Alternative specimens for workplace drug testing. J Anal Toxicol 2001;25:396–399.

401. de la Torre, R, Farre, M, Navarro, M, Pacifici, R, Zuccaro, P, Pichini, S. Clinical pharmacokinetics of amfetamine and related substances: monitoring in conventional and non-conventional matrices. Clin Pharmacokinet 2004;43:157–185.[CrossRef][Web of Science]

402. Pichini, S, Altieri, I, Zuccaro, P, Pacifici, R. Drug monitoring in non-conventional biologic fluids and matrices. Clin Pharmacokinet 1996;30:211–228.

403. Pichini, S, Navarro, M, Pacifici, R, Zuccaro, P, Ortuno, J, Farre, M, et al. Usefulness of sweat testing for the detection of MDMA after a single-dose administration. J Anal Toxicol 2003;27:294–303. [Medline] [Order article via Infotrieve]

404. Samyn, N, De Boeck, G, Verstraete, AG. The use of oral fluid and sweat wipes for the detection of drugs of abuse in drivers. J Forensic Sci 2002;47:1380–1387. [Web of Science][Medline] [Order article via Infotrieve]

405. Haeckel, R, Hanecke, P. The application of saliva, sweat and tear fluids for diagnostic purposes. Ann Biol Clin 1993;50:903–910.

406. Cone, EJ, Hillsgrove, MJ, Jenkins, AJ, Keenan, RM. Sweat testing for heroin, cocaine and metabolites. J Anal Toxicol 1994;18:298–305.

407. Burns, M, Baselt, RC. Monitoring drug use with a sweat patch: an experiment with cocaine. J Anal Toxicol 1995;19:41–48.

408. Kintz, P, Tracqui, A, Mangin, P. Sweat testing in opioid users with a sweat patch. J Anal Toxicol 1996;20:393–397

409. Fay, J, Fogerson, R, Schoendofer, D, Niedbala, RS, Spiehler, V. Detection of methamphetamine in sweat by EIA and GC-MS. J Anal Toxicol 1996;20:398–403.

410. Preston, KL, Huestis, MA, Wong, CJ, Umbricht, A, Goldberger, BA, Cone, EJ. Monitoring cocaine use in substance-abuse-treatment patients by sweat and urine testing. J Anal Toxicol 1999;23:313–322.

411. Huestis, MA, Cone, EJ, Wong, CJ, Umbricht, A, Preston, KL. Monitoring opiate use in substance abuse treatment patients with sweat and urine drug testing. J Anal Toxicol 2000;24:509–521.

412. http://www.nrscience.org/sweat.htm.

413. http://www.webmd.com/skin-problems-and-treatments/features/skin-nutrition.

414. Placzek, M. Journal of Investigative Dermatology, February 2005; vol 124: pp 304–307.

415. Clark, L. The Journal of the American Medical Association, 1996, vol 276: pp 1957–1963.

416. Mitshuishi, T. Journal of Cosmetic Dermatology, April 2004; vol 3. Sha, N.S. Journal of the American Academy of Dermatology, August 2002; vol 47: pp 241–243.

417. Grossman, R. American Journal of Clinical Dermatology 2005; vol 6: pp 39–47.

418. Qing, W. Journal of Clinical Epidemiology, August 1994; vol 47: pp 829–836.

419. Keller, K. Journal of the American Academy of Dermatology, October 1998.

420. Burke, K. Nutrition and Cancer, 1992; vol 17: pp 123–37.

421. Perricone, N. Archives of Gerontology and Geriatrics, July–August 1999; vol 29.

422. Darr, D. Acta Derm Venereol, July 1996; vol 76: pp 264–268.

423. Eberlein–Konig, B. Journal of the American Academy of Dermatology, January 1998; vol 38: pp 45–48.

424. la Ruche, G. Photodermatol Photoimmunol Photomed, December 1991; vol 8: pp 232–235.

425. Naldi, L. British Journal of Dermatology, January 1996. American Academy of Dermatology 2003 Annual Meeting. American Academy of Dermatology.

426. http://en.wikipedia.org/wiki/Dietary_fiber.

427. Katiyar, F, et al. Green Tea and Skin Arch Dermatol. 2000; 136: 989–994.

428. Shaw, N. Green Tea Polyphenols May Be Useful in the Treatment of Androgen-Mediated Skin Disorders Arch Dermatol.2001; 137: 664

429. Santosh, KK, Farrukh A, Anaibelith, P, Mukhtar. Green tea polyphenol (–)-epigallocatechin-3-gallate treatment of human skin inhibits ultraviolet radiation-induced oxidative stress Carcinogenesis, Vol. 22, No. 2, 287–294, February 2001.

430. Wood, JW. Green Tea: What's Brewing? Arch Dermatol.2000; 136: 1051.

431. Toxicological Sciences; Hansen, JM; 82(1):308–317 (2004).

432. American Journal Of Respiratory Cell And Molecular Biology; Das, KC; 17(6):713–726 (1997).

433. British Journal Of Dermatology; Rafferty, TS; 148:1001–1009 (2003).

434. National Research Council: Recommended Dietary Allowances; 10th Edition; Washington, D.C., National Academy of Sciences, 1989.

435. Annual Review Of Nutrition; Bunk, RF; 25:215–235 (2005).

436. The Journal Of Nutrition; Hill, KE; 134(1):157–161 (2004).

437. Clark, LC. Journal Of The American Medical Association; 276(24):1957–1963 (1996).

438. Duffield-Lillico, AJ. Cancer Epidemiology Biomarkers & Prevention; 11(7):630–639 (2002).

439. Taylor, PR. JNCI, Journal Of The National Cancer Institute; 96(6):645–647 (2004).

440. Davis, CD. The Journal Of Nutrition; 133(9):2907–2907 (2003)

441. Davis, CD. The Journal Of Nutrition; 130(12):2903–2909 (2000).

442. Seo, YR. Proceedings Of The National Academy Of Sciences (USA); 99(22):14548–14553 (2002).

443. Longtin, R. JNCI, Journal Of The National Cancer Institute; 95(2):98–100 (2003).

444. Coussens, LM. Nature; 420:860–867 (2002) and Karin, M. Nature Reviews, Immunology; 5(10):749–759 (2005).

445. Kuper, H. Journal Of Internal Medicine; 248(3):171–183 (2000).

446. Jozsef, L. Free Radical Biology & Medicine; 35(9):1018–1027 (2003).

447. Yoon, SO. Journal Of Biological Chemistry; 276(23):20085–20092 (2001).

448. Roussyn, I. Archives Of Biochemistry And Biophysics; 330(1):216–218 (1996).

449. Sies, H. Journal Of Biological Chemistry; 272(44):27812–27817 (1997).

450. Briviba, K. Biochemical Journal; 319(Pt 1):13–15 (1996).

451. Biaglow, JE. Cancer Biology & Therapy; 4(1):6–13 (2005).

452. Journal Of Acquired Immune Deficiency Syndromes And Human Retrovirology; 15(5):370–374 (1997).

453. Beck, MA. The Journal Of Nutrition; 133(5 Suppl 1):1463S–1467S (2003).

454. http://en.wikipedia.org/wiki/Selenium.

455. Broome, CS. The American Journal Of Clinical Nutrition; 80(1):154–162 (2004).

456. Boyne, R. The Journal Of Nutrition; 116(5):816–822 (1986).

457. Davis, CD. The Journal Of Nutrition; 133(5 Suppl 1):1457S–1459S (2003).

458. Sappey, C. Aids Research And Human Retroviruses; 10(11):1451–1461 (1994).

459. Roy, M. Proceedings Of The Society For Experimental Biology And Medicine; 209(4):369–375 (1995).

460. Roy, M. Proceedings Of The Society For Experimental Biology And Medicine; 193(2):143–148 (1990).

461. Kirmedijian-Schumacher, L. Biological Trace Element Research; 41(1–2):115–127 (1994).

462. Stewart, EJ. The Embo Journal; 17(19):5543–5550 (1998).

463. Mitsui, A. Antioxidants & Redox Signaling; 4(2):693–696 (2002).

464. Moskovitz, J. Proceedings Of The National Academy Of Sciences (USA); 100(13):7486–7490(2003).

465. Ruan, H. Proceedings Of The National Academy Of Sciences (USA); 99(5):2748–2753 (2002).

466. Karunasinghe, N. Cancer, Epidemiology, Biomarkers & Prevention; 13(3):391–397 (2004).

467. http://www.cnn.com/2009/HEALTH/expert.q.a/04/10/water.losing.weight.jampolis/index.html.

468. http://wilson.ces.ncsu.edu/index.php?page=news&ci=HEAL+7.

469. Davy, B, et al. Water Consumption Reduces Energy Intake at a Breakfast Meal in Obese Older Adults; Journal of the American Dietetic Association; July 2008.

470. Keller, U, Szinnai, G, Bitz, S, Berneis, K. Effects of changes in hydration on protein, glucose and lipid metabolism in man: impact on health European Journal of Clinical Nutrition (2003) 57, Suppl 2, S69–S74.

471. Arner, P. (1996): Regulation of lipolysis in fat cells. Diab. Rev. 4, 450–463.

472. Baquet, A, Hue, L, Meijer, AJ, Van Woerkom, GM, Plomp, PJAM. (1990): Swelling of rat hepatocytes stimulates glycogen synthesis. J. Biol. Chem. 265, 955–959. | ISI | ChemPort |

473. Berneis, K, Ninnis, R, Häussinger, D, Keller, U. (1999): Effects of hyper- and hypoosmolality on whole-body protein and glucose kinetics in humans. Am. J. Physiol. 276, E188–E195. | PubMed | ChemPort |

474. Beylot, M, Martin, C, Beaufrere, J, Riou, JP, Mornex, R. (1987): Determination of steady state and nonsteady-state glycerol kinetics in humans using deuterium labelled tracer. J. Lipid Res. 28, 414–422.

475. Bilz, S, Ninnis, R, Keller, U. (1999): Effects of hypo-osmolality on whole-body lipolysis in man.Metabolism 48, 472–476.

476. Cobelli, C, Toffolo, G, Bier, D, Nosadini, R. (1987): Models to interpret kinetic data in stable isotope tracer studies. Am. J. Physiol. 253, E551–E564. | PubMed |

477. Finn, J, Lindsay, D, Clark, M, Connolly A, Hill, G. (1996): Progressive cellular dehydration and proteolysis in critically ill patients. Lancet 347, 654–656. | Article | PubMed | ISI | ChemPort |

478. Graf, J, Häussinger, D. (1996): Ion transport in hepatocytes: mechanism and correlation to cell volume, hormone actions and metabolism. J. Hepatol. 24, 53–77.

479. Häussinger, D. (1996): The role of cell hydration for the regulation of cell function. Biochem. J. 313, 697–710.

480. http://www.mayoclinic.com/health/cavities/ds00896/dsection=risk-factors "Cavities/tooth decay".

481. Seal out tooth decay. National Institute of Dental and Craniofacial Research. http://www.nidcr.nih.gov/OralHealth/Topics/ToothDecay/SealOutToothDecay.htm.

482. Fact sheet: Tooth decay. Academy of General Dentistry. http://www.agd.org/public/OralHealthFacts/files/pdfgenerator.aspx?pdf=FS_ToothDecay.pdf&id=.

483. Carmichael, MS, Humbert, R, Dixen, J, Palmisano, G, Greenleaf, W, Davidson, JM. (January 1987). "Plasma oxytocin increases in the human sexual response." The Journal of Clinical Endocrinology

and Metabolism 64 (1): 27–31. http://jcem.endojournals.org/cgi/pmidlookup?view=long&pmid=3782434.

484. Carmichael, MS, Warburton, VL, Dixen, J, Davidson, JM. (February 1994). "Relationships among cardiovascular, muscular, and oxytocin responses during human sexual activity." Archives of Sexual Behavior 23 (1): 59–79.

485. http://www.oxytocin.org/oxytoc/index.html.

486. http://news.bbc.co.uk/2/hi/health/319070.stm.

487. Meston, C. Archives of Sexual Behavior, August 2007; vol 36: pp 477–507.

488. Kosfeld, M. Nature, June 2, 2005; vol 435: pp 673–676.

489. Zak, P. PLoS One, online Nov. 7, 2007.

490. Uryvaev, Y. Bulletin of Experimental Biology and Medicine, November 1996; vol 122: pp 487–489.

491. Leitzmann, M. Journal of the American Medical Association, April 7, 2004; vol 291: pp 1578–1586.

492. Giles, G. BJU International, August 2003; vol 92: pp 211–216.

493. WebMD Medical Reference from Healthwise: "Pelvic Floor (Kegel) Exercises for Urinary Incontinence in Women."

494. American Cancer Society: "Ways of Dealing with Specific Sexual Problems."

495. Lancel, M. Regulatory Peptides, July 15, 2003; vol 114: pp 145–152.

496. WebMD Weight Loss Clinic Feature: "The Dream Diet: Losing Weight While You Sleep."

497. Brody, S. Biological Psychology, February 2006; vol 71: pp 214–222. Brody, S. Biological Psychology, March 2000; vol 52: pp 251–257.

498. Light, KC, et al. "More frequent partner hugs and higher oxytocin levels are linked to lower blood pressure and heart rate in premenopausal women." Biological Psychology, April 2005; vol 69: pp 5–21.

499. Charnetski, CJ, Brennan, FX. Sexual frequency and salivary immunoglobulin A (IgA). Psychological Reports 2004 Jun;94(3 Pt 1):839–44. Data on length of relationship and sexual satisfaction were not related to the group differences.

500. Brody, S. Biological Psychology, February 2006; vol 71: pp 214–222.

501. Brody, S. Biological Psychology, March 2000; vol 52: pp 251–257.

502. Light, K. Biological Psychology, April 2005; vol 69: pp 5–21.

503. Charnetski, C. Psychological Reports, June 2004; vol 94: pp 839–844.

504. Ebrahim, S. Journal of Epidemiology and Community Health, February 2002; vol 56: pp 99–102.

505. Mulhall, J. Journal of Sexual Medicine; online Feb. 8, 2008.

506. Katiyar, S. Journal of Agricultural and Food Chemistry, 2004; vol 52: pp 4026–4037; (use this for blueberries antioxidant amount top four fruits)

507. Carr, AC, Frei, B. Toward a new recommended dietary allowance for vitamin C based on antioxidant and health effects in humans. Am J Clin Nutr. 1999;69(6):1086–1107.

508. Simon, JA, Hudes, ES. Serum ascorbic acid and gallbladder disease prevalence among US adults: the Third National Health and Nutrition Examination Survey (NHANES III). Arch Intern Med. 2000;160(7):931–936.

509. Bruno, RS, Leonard, SW, Atkinson, J, et al. Faster plasma vitamin E disappearance in smokers is normalized by vitamin C supplementation. Free Radic Biol Med. 2006;40(4):689–697.

510. Sauberlich, HE. A history of scurvy and vitamin C. In Packer, L. and Fuchs, J, eds. Vitamin C in health and disease. New York: Marcel Dekker Inc. 1997: pages 1–24.

511. Stephen, R, Utecht, T. Scurvy identified in the emergency department: a case report. J Emerg Med. 2001;21(3):235–237.

512. Weinstein, M, Babyn, P, Zlotkin, S. An orange a day keeps the doctor away: scurvy in the year 2000. Pediatrics. 2001;108(3):E55.

513. Food and Nutrition Board, Institute of Medicine. Vitamin C. Dietary Reference Intakes for Vitamin C, Vitamin E, Selenium, and Carotenoids. Washington D.C.: National Academy Press; 2000:95–185.

514. Ye, Z, Song, H. Antioxidant vitamins intake and the risk of coronary heart disease: meta-analysis of cohort studies. Eur J Cardiovasc Prev Rehabil. 2008;15(1):26–34.

515. Losonczy, KG, Harris, TB, Havlik, RJ. Vitamin E and vitamin C supplement use and risk of all-cause and coronary heart disease mortality in older persons: the Established Populations for Epidemiologic Studies of the Elderly. Am J Clin Nutr. 1996;64(2):190–196.

516. Kushi, LH, Folsom, AR, Prineas, RJ, Mink, PJ, Wu, Y, Bostick, RM. Dietary antioxidant vitamins and death from coronary heart disease in postmenopausal women. N Engl J Med. 1996;334(18):1156–1162.

517. McCormick, DB. Vitamin B6. In: Bowman BA, Russell RM, eds. Present Knowledge in Nutrition. Vol. I. Washington, D.C.: International Life Sciences Institute; 2006:269–277.

518. Leklem, JE. Vitamin B6. In: Machlin L, ed. Handbook of Vitamins. New York: Marcel Dekker Inc; 1991:341–378.

519. Dakshinamurti, S, Dakshinamurti, K. Vitamin B6. In: Zempleni J, Rucker RB, McCormick DB, Suttie JW, eds. Handbook of Vitamins. 4th ed. New York: CRC Press (Taylor & Fracis Group); 2007:315–359.

520. Leklem, JE. Vitamin B6. In: Shils M, Olson JA, Shike M, Ross AC, eds. Modern Nutrition in Health and Disease. 9th ed. Baltimore: Williams & Wilkins; 1999:413–422.

521. Mackey, AD, Davis, SR, Gregory, JF, 3rd. Vitamin B6. In: Shils ME, Shike M, Ross AC, Caballero B, Cousins RJ, eds. Modern Nutrition in Health and Disease. 10th ed. Philadelphia: Lippincott Williams & Wilkins; 2006:452–461.

522. Hansen, CM, Leklem, JE, Miller, LT. Vitamin B-6 status of women with a constant intake of vitamin B-6 changes with three levels of dietary protein. J Nutr. 1996;126(7):1891–1901.

523. Food and Nutrition Board, Institute of Medicine. Vitamin B6. Dietary Reference Intakes: Thiamin, Riboflavin, Niacin, Vitamin B6, Vitamin B12, Pantothenic Acid, Biotin, and Choline. Washington D.C.: National Academies Press; 1998:150–195.

524. Boushey, CJ, Beresford, SA, Omenn, GS, Motulsky, AG. A quantitative assessment of plasma homocysteine as a risk factor for vascular disease. Probable benefits of increasing folic acid intakes. JAMA. 1995;274(13):1049–1057.

525. Rimm, EB, Willett, WC, Hu, FB, et al. Folate and vitamin B6 from diet and supplements in relation to risk of coronary heart disease among women. JAMA. 1998;279(5):359–364.

526. Folsom, AR, Nieto, FJ, McGovern, PG, et al. Prospective study of coronary heart disease incidence in relation to fasting total homocysteine, related genetic polymorphisms, and B vitamins: the Atherosclerosis Risk in Communities (ARIC) study. Circulation. 1998;98(3):204–210.

527. Robinson, K, Arheart, K, Refsum, H, et al. Low circulating folate and vitamin B6 concentrations: risk factors for stroke, peripheral vascular disease, and coronary artery disease. European COMAC Group. Circulation. 1998;97(5):437–443.

528. Robinson, K, Mayer, EL, Miller, DP, et al. Hyperhomocysteinemia and low pyridoxal phosphate. Common and independent reversible risk factors for coronary artery disease. Circulation. 1995;92(10):2825–2830.

529. Lin, PT, Cheng, CH, Liaw, YP, Lee, BJ, Lee, TW, Huang, YC. Low pyridoxal 5'-phosphate is associated with increased risk of coronary artery disease. Nutrition. 2006;22(11–12):1146–1151.

530. Ubbink, JB, Vermaak, WJ, van der Merwe, A, Becker, PJ, Delport, R, Potgieter, HC. Vitamin requirements for the treatment of hyperhomocysteinemia in humans. J Nutr. 1994;124(10):1927–1933.

531. Meydani, SN, Ribaya-Mercado, JD, Russell, RM, Sahyoun, N, Morrow, FD, Gershoff, SN. Vitamin B-6 deficiency impairs interleukin 2

production and lymphocyte proliferation in elderly adults. Am J Clin Nutr. 1991;53(5):1275–1280.

532. Talbott, MC, Miller, LT, Kerkvliet, NI. Pyridoxine supplementation: effect on lymphocyte responses in elderly persons. Am J Clin Nutr. 1987;46(4):659–664.

533. Holick, MF. Vitamin D: importance in the prevention of cancers, type 1 diabetes, heart disease, and osteoporosis. Am J Clin Nutr. 2004;79(3):362–371.

534. Armas, LA, Hollis, BW, Heaney, RP. Vitamin D2 is much less effective than vitamin D3 in humans. J Clin Endocrinol Metab. 2004;89(11):5387–5391.

535. Holick, MF. Vitamin D: A millenium perspective. J Cell Biochem. 2003;88(2):296–307.

536. Sutton, AL, MacDonald, PN. Vitamin D: more than a "bone-a-fide" hormone. Mol Endocrinol. 2 003;17(5):777–791.

537. Guyton, KZ, Kensler, TW, Posner, GH. Vitamin D and vitamin D analogs as cancer chemopreventive agents. Nutr Rev. 2003;61(7):227–238.

538. DeLuca, HF. Overview of general physiologic features and functions of vitamin D. Am J Clin Nutr. 2004;80(6 Suppl):1689S–1696S.

539. Lin, R, White, JH. The pleiotropic actions of vitamin D. Bioessays. 2004;26(1):21–28.

540. Hayes, CE, Nashold, FE, Spach, KM, Pedersen, LB. The immunological functions of the vitamin D endocrine system. Cell Mol Biol. 2003;49(2):277–300.

541. Griffin, MD, Xing, N, Kumar, R. Vitamin D and its analogs as regulators of immune activation and antigen presentation. Annu Rev Nutr. 2003;23:117–145.

542. Food and Nutrition Board, Institute of Medicine. Vitamin D. Dietary Reference Intakes: Calcium, Phosphorus, Magnesium, Vitamin D, and Fluoride. Washington D.C.: National Academies Press; 1999:250–287.

543. Wagner, CL, Greer, FR, and the Section on Breastfeeding and Committee on Nutrition. Prevention of rickets and vitamin D deficiency in infants, children, and adolescents. American Academy of Pediatrics. 2008;122(5):1142–1152. Available at: http://www.aap.org/new/VitaminDreport.pdf.

544. Bischoff-Ferrari, HA, Giovannucci, E, Willett, WC, Dietrich, T, Dawson-Hughes, B. Estimation of optimal serum concentrations of 25-hydroxyvitamin D for multiple health outcomes. Am J Clin Nutr. 2006;84(1):18–28.

545. Heaney, RP. Vitamin D: how much do we need, and how much is too much? Osteoporos Int. 2000;11(7):553–555.

546. Hollis, BW. Circulating 25-hydroxyvitamin D levels indicative of vitamin D sufficiency: implications for establishing a new effective dietary intake recommendation for vitamin D. J Nutr. 2005;135(2):317–322.

547. Vieth, R. Why the optimal requirement for Vitamin D3 is probably much higher than what is officially recommended for adults. J Steroid Biochem Mol Biol. 2004;89–90(1–5):575–579.

548. Lips, P, Hosking, D, Lippuner, K, et al. The prevalence of vitamin D inadequacy amongst women with osteoporosis: an international epidemiological investigation. J Intern Med. 2006;260(3):245–254.

549. Trumbo, PR. Pantothenic acid. In: Shils ME, Shike M, Ross AC, Caballero B, Cousins RJ, eds. Modern Nutrition in Health and Disease. 10th ed. Philadelphia: Lippincott Williams & Wilkins; 2006:462–469.

550. Tahiliani, AG, Beinlich, CJ. Pantothenic acid in health and disease. Vitam Horm. 1991;46:165–228.

551. Brody, T. Nutritional Biochemistry. 2nd ed. San Diego: Academic Press; 1999.

552. Plesofsky-Vig, N. Pantothenic acid. In: Shils ME, Olson JA, Shike M, Ross AC, eds. Modern Nutrition in Health and Disease. 9th ed. Philadelphia: Lippincott Williams & Wilkins; 1999:423–432.

553. Bender, DA. Optimum nutrition: thiamin, biotin and pantothenate. Proc Nutr Soc. 1999;58(2):427–433.

554. Hodges, RE, Ohlson, MA, Bean, WB. Pantothenic acid deficiency in man. J Clin Invest. 1958;37:1642–1657.

555. Fry, PC, Fox, HM, Tao, HG. Metabolic response to a pantothenic acid deficient diet in humans. J Nutr Sci Vitaminol (Tokyo). 1976;22(4):339–346.

556. Food and Nutrition Board, Institute of Medicine. Pantothenic acid. Dietary Reference Intakes: Thiamin, Riboflavin, Niacin, Vitamin B-6, Vitamin B-12, Pantothenic Acid, Biotin, and Choline. Washington, D.C.: National Academy Press; 1998:357–373.

557. Food and Nutrition Board, Institute of Medicine. Biotin. Dietary Reference Intakes: Thiamin, Riboflavin, Niacin, Vitamin B6, Vitamin B12, Pantothenic Acid, Biotin, and Choline. Washington, D.C.: National Academy Press; 1998:374–389.

558. Mock, DM. Biotin. In: Shils ME, Olson JA, Shike M, Ross AC, eds. Modern Nutrition in Health and Disease. 9th ed. Baltimore: Lippincott Williams & Wilkins; 1999:459–466.

559. Chapman-Smith, A, Cronan, JE, Jr. Molecular biology of biotin attachment to proteins. J Nutr. 1999;129(2S Suppl):477S–484S.

560. Zempleni, J, Mock, DM. Biotin biochemistry and human requirements. 1999; volume 10: pages 128–138. J Nutr. Biochem. 1999;10:128–138.

561. Hymes, J, Wolf, B. Human biotinidase isn't just for recycling biotin. J Nutr. 1999;129(2S Suppl):485S–489S.

562. Zempleni, J, Mock, DM. Marginal biotin deficiency is teratogenic. Proc Soc Exp Biol Med. 2000;223(1):14–21.

563. Kothapalli, N, Camporeale, G, Kueh, A, et al. Biological functions of biotinylated histones. J Nutr Biochem. 2005;16(7):446–448.

564. Mock, DM. Biotin. In: Shils ME, Shike M, Ross AC, Caballero B, Cousins RJ, eds. Modern Nutrition in Health and Disease. 10th ed. Baltimore: Lippincott Williams & Wilkins; 2006:482–497.

565. Brody, T. Nutritional Biochemistry. 2nd ed. San Diego: Academic Press; 1999.

566. Cervantes-Laurean, D, McElvaney, NG, Moss, J. Niacin. In: Shils M, Olson JA, Shike M, Ross AC, eds. Modern Nutrition in Health and Disease. 9th ed. Baltimore: Williams & Wilkins; 1999:401–411.

567. Jacob, R, Swenseid, M. Niacin. In: Ziegler EE, Filer LJ, eds. Present Knowledge in Nutrition. 7th ed. Washington D.C: ILSI Press; 1996:185–190.

568. Jacobson, MK, Jacobson, EL. Discovering new ADP-ribose polymer cycles: protecting the genome and more. Trends Biochem Sci. 1999;24(11):415–417.

569. Park, YK, Sempos, CT, Barton, CN, Vanderveen, JE, Yetley, EA. Effectiveness of food fortification in the United States: the case of pellagra. Am J Public Health. 2000;90(5):727–738.

570. Gregory, JF, 3rd. Nutritional Properties and significance of vitamin glycosides. Annu Rev Nutr. 1998;18:277–296.

571. Fu, CS, Swendseid, ME, Jacob, RA, McKee, RW. Biochemical markers for assessment of niacin status in young men: levels of erythrocyte niacin coenzymes and plasma tryptophan. J Nutr. 1989;119(12):1949–1955.

572. Food and Nutrition Board, Institute of Medicine. Niacin. Dietary Reference Intakes: Thiamin, Riboflavin, Niacin, Vitamin B6, Vitamin B12, Pantothenic Acid, Biotin, and Choline. Washington, D.C.: National Academy Press; 1998:123–149.

573. Jacobson, EL, Jacobson, MK. Tissue NAD as a biochemical measure of niacin status in humans. Methods Enzymol. 1997;280:221–230.

574. Jacobson, EL, Shieh, WM, Huang, AC. Mapping the role of NAD metabolism in prevention and treatment of carcinogenesis. Mol Cell Biochem. 1999;193(1–2):69–74.

575. Food and Nutrition Board, Institute of Medicine. Riboflavin. Dietary Reference Intakes: Thiamin, Riboflavin, Niacin, Vitamin B6, Vitamin

B12, Pantothenic Acid, Biotin, and Choline. Washington D.C.: National Academy Press; 1998:87–122.

576. Brody, T. Nutritional Biochemistry. 2nd ed. San Diego: Academic Press; 1999.

577. McCormick, DB. Riboflavin. In: Shils M, Olson JA, Shike M, Ross AC, eds. Modern Nutrition in Health and Disease. 9th ed. Baltimore: Williams & Wilkins; 1999:391–399.

578. Powers, HJ. Current knowledge concerning optimum nutritional status of riboflavin, niacin and pyridoxine. Proc Nutr Soc. 1999;58(2):435–440.

579. Rivlin, RS. Riboflavin. In: Ziegler EE, Filer LJ, eds. Present Knowledge in Nutrition. 7th ed. Washington D.C.: ILSI Press; 1996:167–173.

580. Bohles, H. Antioxidative vitamins in prematurely and maturely born infants. Int J Vitam Nutr Res. 1997;67(5):321–328.

581. McCormick, DB. Two interconnected B vitamins: riboflavin and pyridoxine. Physiol Rev. 1989;69(4):1170–1198.

582. Madigan, SM, Tracey, F, McNulty, H, et al. Riboflavin and vitamin B-6 intakes and status and biochemical response to riboflavin supplementation in free-living elderly people. Am J Clin Nutr. 1998;68(2):389–395.

583. Lowik, MR, van den Berg, H, Kistemaker, C, Brants, HA, Brussaard, JH. Interrelationships between riboflavin and vitamin B6 among elderly people (Dutch Nutrition Surveillance System). Int J Vitam Nutr Res. 1994;64(3):198–203.

584. Jacques, PF, Bostom, AG, Wilson, PW, Rich, S, Rosenberg, IH, Selhub, J. Determinants of plasma total homocysteine concentration in the Framingham Offspring cohort. Am J Clin Nutr. 2001;73(3):613–621.

585. Brody, T. Nutritional Biochemistry. 2nd ed. San Diego: Academic Press; 1999.

586. Carmel, R. Cobalamin (Vitamin B-12). In: Shils ME, Shike M, Ross AC, Caballero B, Cousins RJ, eds. Modern Nutrition in Health and Disease. Philadelphia: Lippincott Williams & Wilkins;2006:482–497.

587. Shane, B. Folic acid, vitamin B-12, and vitamin B-6. In: Stipanuk M, ed. Biochemical and Physiological Aspects of Human Nutrition. Philadelphia: W.B. Saunders Co.; 2000:483–518.

588. Baik, HW, Russell, RM. Vitamin B12 deficiency in the elderly. Annu Rev Nutr. 1999;19:357–377.

589. Herbert, V. Vitamin B-12. In: Ziegler EE, Filer LJ, eds. Present Knowledge in Nutrition. 7th ed. Washington D.C.: ILSI Press; 1996:191–205.

590. Food and Nutrition Board, Institute of Medicine. Vitamin B12. Dietary Reference Intakes: Thiamin, Riboflavin, Niacin, Vitamin B6, Vitamin

B12, Pantothenic Acid, Biotin, and Choline. Washington D.C.: National Academy Press; 1998:306–356.

591. Kuzminski, AM, Del Giacco, EJ, Allen, RH, Stabler, SP, Lindenbaum, J. Effective treatment of cobalamin deficiency with oral cobalamin. Blood. 1998;92(4):1191–1198.

592. Lederle, FA. Oral cobalamin for pernicious anemia. Medicine's best kept secret? JAMA. 1991;265(1):94–95.

593. http://lpi.oregonstate.edu.

594. Groff, JL. Advanced Nutrition and Human Metabolism. 2nd ed. St Paul: West Publishing; 1995.

595. Ross, AC. Vitamin A and retinoids. In: Shils M, ed. Nutrition in Health and Disease. 9th ed. Baltimore: Williams & Wilkins; 1999:305–327.

596. Semba, RD. The role of vitamin A and related retinoids in immune function. Nutr Rev. 1998;56(1 Pt 2):S38–48.

597. Semba, RD. Impact of vitamin A on immunity and infection in developing countries. In: Bendich A, Decklebaum RJ, eds. Preventive Nutrition: The Comprehensive Guide for Health Professionals. 2nd ed. Totowa: Humana Press Inc; 2001:329–346.

598. McCullough, F, et al. The effect of vitamin A on epithelial integrity. Proceedings of the Nutrition Society. 1999; volume 58: pages 289–293.

599. Solomons, NW. Vitamin A and carotenoids. In: Bowman BA, Russell RM, eds. Present Knowledge in Nutrition. 8th ed. Washington D.C.: ILSI Press; 2001:127–145.

600. Lynch, SR. Interaction of iron with other nutrients. Nutr Rev. 1997;55(4):102–110.

601. Russell, RM. The vitamin A spectrum: from deficiency to toxicity. Am J Clin Nutr. 2000;71(4):878–884.

602. Brody, T. Nutritional Biochemistry. 2nd ed. San Diego: Academic Press; 1999.

603. Christian, P, West, KP, Jr. Interactions between zinc and vitamin A: an update. Am J Clin Nutr. 1998;68(2 Suppl):435S–441S.

604. Atwater, WO. The Potential Energy of Food. The Chemistry and Economy of Food. III. Century1887; 34:397–405.

605. Berlin, CM, Schimke, RT. Influence of turnover rates on the responses of enzymes to cortisone. Mol Pharmacol. 1:149, 1965.

606. Kleiber, M. The Fire of Life, An Introduction to Animal Energetics. New York: Huntington: Robert Kreiger; 1975.

607. Hargrove, JL, Schmidt, FH. The role of mRNA and protein stability in gene expression.FASEB J. 3:2360, 1989.

608. Berman, M, Weiss, MF, Shawn, E. Some formal approaches to the analysis of kinetic data in terms of linear compartmental systems. Biophys J. 2:289, 1962.

609. Wastney, ME, House, WA, et al. Kinetics of zinc metabolism: Variation with diet, genetics and disease. J. Nutr. 130:1355S, 2000.

610. Diwadkar-Navsariwala, V, Novotny, JA, Gustin, DM, et al. A physiological pharmacokinetic model describing the disposition of lycopene in healthy men. J. Lipid Res. 44: 1927, 2003.

611. Gallaher, EJ. Biological System Dynamics: From Personal Discovery to Universal Application. Simulation. 66:243, 1996

612. Das, SK, Gilhooly, CH, Golden, JK, et al. Long-term effects of 2 energy-restricted diets differing in glycemic load on dietary adherence, body composition, and metabolism in CALERIE: a 1-y randomized controlled trial. Am J Clin Nutr. 85:1023, 2007.

613. http://www.nytimes.com/2009/10/11/magazine/11Calories-t.html?fta=y.

614. http://news.sciencemag.org/sciencenow/2009/07/09-01.html "Calorie-Counting Monkeys Live Longer."

615. http://www.nytimes.com/2009/07/10/science/10aging.html

616. http://www.nytimes.com/2006/11/07/science/07drug.html?fta=y Aging Drugs: Hardest Test Is Still Ahead.

617. http://www.nytimes.com/2009/09/29/science/29aging.html?ref=caloric_restriction "Quest for a Long Life Gains Scientific Respect/"

618. http://www.nytimes.com/2007/05/03/health/03gene.html Gene Links Longevity and Diet, Scientists Say.

619. http://en.wikipedia.org/wiki/FOX_proteins.

620. van der Horst, A, Burgering, BM. (June 2007). "Stressing the role of Fox proteins in lifespan and disease." Nat. Rev. Mol. Cell Biol. 8 (6): 440–50.

621. Hannenhalli, S, Kaestner, KH. The evolution of Fox genes and their role in development and disease Nature Reviews Genetics 10, 233–240 (1 April 2009) | doi:10.1038/nrg2523.

622. Keys, A, Brozek, J, Henschel, A, Mickelsen O, Taylor, HL. The Biology of Human Starvation (2 volumes), University of Minnesota Press, 1950.

623. Tucker, T. The Great Starvation Experiment: The Heroic Men Who Starved so That Millions Could Live, Free Press, A Division of Simon & Schuster, Inc., New York, New York, ISBN 978-0-7432-7030-4, 2006.

624. Kalm, LM, Semba, RD. "They Starved So That Others Be Better Fed: Remembering Ancel Keys and the Minnesota Experiment," Journal of Nutrition, Vol. 135, June 2005, 1347–1352.

625. Chaput, JP, Tremblay, A. Adaptive Reduction in Thermogenesis and Resistance to Lose Fat in Obese Men. The British Journal of Nutrition. 102:488, 2009.

626. Leibel, RL, Rosenbaum, M, Hirsch, J. Changes in energy expenditure resulting from altered body weight. N Engl J Med. 332:621, 1995.

627. Ganley, T. Dodging the Dreaded Plateau: Confusing Your Muscles to Make Fitness Gains. Tampa Bay Wellness. Tampa, Florida. June 2008.

Index

I

Ideal weight range, 140–143
Immune system, 3–4, 20, 30, 126–127, 161, 164
Immunoglobulin A (IgA), 126, 128
Insoluble fiber, 42, 44
Insulin resistance, 80, 100
International Forgiveness Institute, 16
Intimacy, 127
Iodine, 55
Iron, 56

K

Kegel exercises, 127
Kidneys
    detoxification and, 189, 190, 191, 193–196
    high-protein diets and, xviii, 84–85, 145
    kidney disease, xviii, xxvi–xxvii, 63, 84, 85, 145, 190, 194–196
    soft drinks and, 63
    water and, 9–10, 197

L

Large intestine. See Colon
Laughter, 30
The Laws of Temperaments (Maimonides), 117–118
LDL cholesterol, 43, 85, 96, 97, 98, 100, 144, 163, 167, 185
Leptin, 12
Lignan, 182
Limbic system, 27–28
Linoleic acids, 45, 46, 96, 99
Linolenic acids, 45, 46, 99
Lipid peroxidation, 112
Liposuction, xxvii
Liver, 10, 64, 84, 189, 190–191
Love, 1–2, 3–4, 15

L.O.V.E. Diet Program
    about, xxiii, 144–145
    composition of, 72–77, 137
    determining calories, 149–151
    food groups for, 69–71
    rate your own plate, 155–156
    weight loss contract, 146, 152–154
    worksheet for, 147–148
    See also Ten Commandments
Lovemaking. See Sex
Low-carb diets, xxv–xxvii
Low-glycemic index foods, 40, 90–94, 100, 138
Lutein, 58, 163, 166, 178, 182, 184
Lycopene, 58, 163, 167, 178, 182, 184

M

Macronutrients, 39, 81
Magnesium, 56
Maimonides, xv, xxiii, 117–118
Manganese, 56
Massage therapy, 25
Meditation, 5, 6–7, 14
Memory and emotion, 17
Menopause, 126
Metabolism, 65, 82, 87–89, 223
Micronutrients, 39, 81
Mind, nourishment of, 29–33
Mind-body connection, 29
Mindscape, 13–14
Minerals, 8, 39, 54–57, 69, 101
Minnesota Starvation Experiment, 221
Monounsaturated fats, 73, 96–99
Mood, 30
Muscle confusion technique, 223–224
My Optimum Plate, 72–77
MyPlate icon, 71–72

Printed in the United States
By Bookmasters